Sleep Smarter

Unlocking the Secrets to Restful
Nights and Energized Days

By
Dr. Sarah Nightingale

Sleep Smarter

Unlocking the Secrets to Restful
Nights and Energized Days

Table of Contents

Introduction

M any of us have experienced the bane of a sleepless night, only to drag ourselves through the next day with a foggy mind and irritability. Whether you're a busy professional working against tight deadlines or a student burning the midnight oil, sleep often becomes a casualty. Yet, what's often underappreciated is just how vital sleep is to our overall health and well-being. Indeed, the quality of our lives heavily leans on the quality of our sleep.

Even though sleep might seem trivial compared to the endless tasks awaiting us, it serves as a pillar of good health, alongside diet and exercise. Whether you're looking to excel at work, improve your studies, or just feel better overall, sleep is the magic bullet that can elevate every aspect of your life. In this book, we're diving deep to help you reclaim what might be the most underrated part of your day.

Let's be real: sacrificing sleep isn't a sustainable solution. Many people view sleep as expendable, something that can be trimmed away to make more room for a busy schedule. In reality, this can lead to a downward spiral of health issues, cognitive decline, and even emotional instability (Walker, 2017). The purpose of this book is not to guilt-trip you into better sleeping habits but to arm you with the knowledge and tools needed to make informed choices about your sleep.

Consider this: your body literally runs on sleep. From stabilizing moods to improving memory, the benefits are multifaceted. But it's not just about racking up hours; it's about the quality of those hours, too. Poor sleep can negatively impact almost every biological function, yet many of us are stuck in a cycle of subpar rest. This book aims to break you free from this damaging loop.

First, we'll explore why sleep is so critical. You'll discover the compelling connections between sleep and health, how it affects cognitive function, and the surprising ways your body uses sleep to rejuvenate. We'll debunk common myths and provide science-based insights you can apply immediately to enhance your sleep quality. We'll walk you through complex biological mechanisms, but in a way that's both engaging and easy to grasp (Huffington, 2016).

Next, we venture into the fascinating world of sleep biology. Imagine peeking into the intricate dance of your sleep cycles and understanding the stages your body transitions through each night. Knowledge is power, and grasping these basics will give you a solid foundation to tackle your sleep issues head-on.

Of course, we can't ignore the myriad sleep disorders that plague many of us. From insomnia to sleep apnea and beyond, understanding the nuances of these conditions is the first step toward finding effective solutions. Rest assured, we've distilled the latest research and expert opinions to offer practical advice that you can implement without overwhelming yourself.

There's also a lot of misinformation out there. How many times have you heard someone say they can 'catch up' on sleep over the weekend? Or that a nightcap will help them sleep better? Spoiler alert: these are myths, and we'll debunk them with hard science. Disentangling fact from fiction is crucial for your journey towards better sleep.

Your environment also plays a pivotal role in how well you sleep. From your bedroom setup to the optimal temperature and lighting conditions, we'll guide you through creating a sleep oasis that sets the stage for optimal rest.

Ever wondered how your diet affects your sleep? Nutrition and sleep are intricately linked. We'll demystify which foods can help you drift off easily and which ones to avoid. Plus, learn about the perils of technology on sleep and how to mitigate its disruptive effects.

Stress is often an inescapable part of modern life, but it doesn't have to sabotage your sleep. We'll introduce you to relaxation techniques, mindfulness practices, and even specific types of exercise that can significantly improve your sleep quality.

Establishing a consistent sleep routine might sound basic, but it's one of the most effective ways to enhance sleep quality. From pre-sleep rituals to the power of consistency, we'll walk you through actionable steps that can make a world of difference.

For those considering sleep aids, we'll look at both over-the-counter options and natural alternatives, providing an objective view to help you make informed decisions. Plus, if you're a shift worker or a frequent traveler, we've got tailored advice to help you navigate the unique challenges you face in getting quality sleep.

By the time we wrap up, you'll not only understand the importance of sleep but also have a toolkit of strategies to transform how you rest. We're not just aiming for more sleep here; we're aiming for better sleep. Quality over quantity. How you sleep tonight can shape your tomorrow, and it all begins with understanding and optimizing your sleep today. So, turn the page and let's begin this sleep revolution together.

Chapter 1:
The Importance of Sleep

Getting a good night's sleep isn't just about feeling rested; it's foundational to nearly every aspect of our well-being. Whether you're striving for career success, academic excellence, or simply looking to enhance your overall quality of life, prioritizing sleep is essential. Scientific studies repeatedly show that sleep plays a critical role in physical health, mental clarity, emotional stability, and cognitive function (Hirshkowitz et al., 2015). When we're well-rested, we're more productive, creative, and resilient. Conversely, chronic sleep deprivation can lead to a host of problems, including increased risk of chronic diseases like diabetes and heart disease, impaired judgment, and susceptibility to mood disorders like anxiety and depression (Watson et al., 2015). Given the impact of sleep on our daily lives, it's time to start treating it as the non-negotiable pillar of health that it truly is.

Sleep and Health

Sleep is not just a state of rest; it's a crucial pillar of health and well-being. Imagine sleep as the nightly maintenance crew that comes in to repair, rejuvenate, and energize your body and mind. It holds fundamental importance across various facets of life, impacting everything from immune function and heart health to mental wellness and longevity.

For starters, let's talk about how sleep impacts your heart. A growing body of research highlights a strong connection between poor sleep and cardiovascular diseases. Studies have shown that those who consistently get inadequate sleep are at a higher risk for high blood pressure, stroke, and heart attacks (Grandner & Buxton, 2013). When you sleep, your heart rate and blood pressure fall, promoting heart health. But disrupting this restorative period can lead to sustained increased blood pressure throughout the day.

In close relation to heart health is the functioning of your immune system. It's like the knight in shining armor, defending your body against invaders. However, neglecting to give your knight time to rest can prove disastrous. During sleep, your immune system releases proteins called cytokines, some of which are essential for fighting off infections and inflammation. Chronic sleep deprivation decreases the production of these protective proteins, thereby weakening your immune defenses (Durmer & Dinges, 2005).

Weight management and metabolic health are also tightly linked with sleep quality. When you don't get enough rest, two critical hormones—ghrelin and leptin—get thrown off balance. Ghrelin, the "hunger hormone," spikes, causing you to feel hungrier, while leptin, which signals fullness, diminishes. This imbalance can lead to increased calorie intake and, subsequently, weight gain (Taheri et al., 2004). It's not just about feeling sleepy during the day; it's about increasing your risk for conditions like obesity and type 2 diabetes.

Ever notice how your bad mood hangs around longer when you're running on fumes? That's not a coincidence. Emotionally, sleep acts as a reset button. It's during REM sleep that the brain processes emotional experiences, helping to maintain emotional stability. Chronic sleep deprivation can lead to mood swings, anxiety, and even depression. In fact, insomniacs are ten times more likely to suffer from clinical depression than those who sleep well (Ford & Kamerow, 1989).

Cognitive health ties in very closely with emotional well-being. Memory consolidation, problem-solving, and learning abilities are all enhanced during sleep. Think of sleep as uploading the day's experiences to your brain's hard drive. Interrupt that process, and you essentially disrupt your learning and memory creation mechanisms (Rasch & Born, 2013). Whether you're a student cramming for exams or a professional aiming for peak performance, deprioritizing sleep can cost you dearly in cognitive function.

But let's not just focus on the negatives. The benefits of good sleep extend to some of the most delightful aspects of life, such as skin health. During sleep, blood flow to the skin increases, collagen rebuilds, and damage from UV exposure is repaired. Conversely, lack of sleep accelerates the aging process, leading to wrinkles, dull complexion, and dark circles under the eyes. It's literally a beauty sleep.

Sleep also has a role in longevity. Studies have found that both too little and too much sleep can negatively affect lifespan. A meta-analysis concluded that consistently sleeping less than six hours a night or more than nine hours is associated with an increased risk of death from any cause (Cappuccio et al., 2010). Thus, striking that perfect balance in sleep duration is crucial for a long, healthy life.

During these challenging times, emotional resilience is more crucial than ever. And guess what? Sleep nourishes your ability to cope with stress and adversity. When you're well-rested, you're better equipped to tackle the ups and downs life throws at you. You're not just reacting to situations but responding thoughtfully. Chronic sleep deprivation, on the other hand, places you in a constant state of heightened alertness—leaving you less adaptable and more prone to stress.

Did you know sleep deprivation could also affect your social life? When you're exhausted, you're less likely to be your most charismatic self, less engaged in conversations, and generally less approachable. You might not think it, but poor sleep can alienate you from social interactions, affecting your relationships in ways you might not immediately recognize.

The importance of sleep extends to general body wellness too. During deep sleep stages, growth hormone is released, aiding in muscle repair and growth, and tissue regeneration. If you're into sports or fitness, neglecting sleep can hamper your athletic performance, increasing your risk of injury and delaying recovery times.

Finally, let's look at how sleep interacts with substance use. Sleep deprivation increases the likelihood of risk-taking behaviors, including substance abuse. Lack of sleep alters the reward pathways in the brain, making you more susceptible to addictive behaviors. It's a vicious cycle: substance use further disrupts sleep, exacerbating the problem.

In conclusion, sleep is a multifaceted gem in the crown of health and wellness, exerting influence over cardiovascular health, immune function, weight management, cognitive performance, emotional stability, skin health, and even social interactions. Understanding and prioritizing your sleep can dramatically enhance your quality of life. It's not just about the quantity of sleep but the quality too. Listen to your body and treat sleep as the powerful, restorative force it truly is.

Sleep and Cognitive Function

Sleep and cognitive function are deeply intertwined, more than most of us realize. It's not just about feeling rested; it's literally about how your brain works. Ever wondered why your thoughts get fuzzy or why multitasking feels impossible after a bad night's sleep? That's your brain crying out for more shut-eye. Cognitive function encompasses attention, memory, problem-solving, and decision-making—all of which take a hit when you're sleep-deprived.

Think about it: during sleep, your brain is incredibly active. There's a lot going on behind the scenes, like memory consolidation and toxin removal (Xie et al., 2013). When you're asleep, your brain is busy packaging up the information from the day and solidifying memories. It's like clearing out your email inbox, organizing your desktop, and installing critical software updates—all while you snooze. Without sufficient sleep, these processes don't work properly, and you're left feeling foggy and forgetful.

One of the most well-known processes affected by sleep is memory consolidation. Studies show that sufficient sleep is crucial for both declarative memory (facts and knowledge) and procedural memory (skills and tasks) (Walker & Stickgold, 2004). When you pull an all-nighter, you're more likely to forget what you just learned or make mistakes on tasks and projects. You might cram for a test and hope for the best, but science suggests you would be better off getting a good night's sleep.

Attention and focus are also significantly affected by sleep quality. Ever tried to focus on a deadline-driven project after a sleepless night? It's a struggle, right? Sleep deprivation makes selective attention an enormous challenge (Lim & Dinges, 2010). You might find yourself easily distracted, unable to keep your thoughts aligned, and your productivity plummets. Sufficient sleep enables your prefrontal cortex, the area of the brain responsible for complex cognitive behavior and decision-making, to function efficiently. Without it, you're operating on cognitive fumes.

Decision-making skills decline significantly without adequate sleep. Researchers have found that sleep deprivation affects the way we evaluate risk and reward, often leading us to make less rational decisions (Venkatraman et al., 2007). This isn't just about big life decisions; it affects everyday choices too. Poor sleep can change your outlook, making you more impulsive and less able to consider long-term consequences. Not exactly a recipe for success.

Problem-solving is another cognitive area that takes a hit when we don't get enough sleep. A study has shown that sleep improves performance on tasks requiring creative problem-solving and insight (Wagner et al., 2004). When you're sleep-deprived, your ability to think outside the box diminishes. You may find yourself stuck in a loop, unable to find innovative solutions to problems that would otherwise seem straightforward with a well-rested mind.

Even social cognition isn't immune to the ravages of sleep deprivation. It's the part of our cognition that affects how we understand and interact with others. Being sleep-deprived can lead to a decrease in emotional empathy and the ability to correctly interpret social cues (Goldstein & Walker, 2014). This can be a big problem if your job requires you to be in constant communication with others or if you're working in a team setting. Misinterpreting someone's mood or failing to respond appropriately could lead to conflicts and misunderstandings.

What's critical to understand is that these cognitive functions don't just operate in isolation. They're interconnected. Poor attention leads to poorer memory retention, bad decision-making affects problem-solving, and impaired social cognition can escalate your stress levels, spiraling further cognitive decline. It's like a cognitive domino effect that all circles back to one culprit: lack of sleep.

To optimize cognitive function, it's not just about the quantity of sleep but also the quality. Scientists recommend aiming for 7-9 hours of sleep per night with a focus on achieving restorative stages of sleep, such as REM (rapid eye movement) and deep sleep (Hirshkowitz et al., 2015). REM sleep is particularly important for memory consolidation and emotional regulation. If you ever wonder why you feel more emotionally volatile after a poor night's sleep, it's because you haven't had enough REM sleep.

In practical terms, improving your sleep quality can have substantial benefits for cognitive function. For example, establishing a regular sleep schedule, creating a relaxing bedtime routine, and ensuring your sleep environment is conducive to rest are all proven methods to enhance sleep (National Sleep Foundation, 2020). Practices such as avoiding screens before bed and reducing caffeine intake can also make a significant difference.

Moreover, understanding the importance of sleep and taking actionable steps isn't just a personal triumph; it can improve the broader dynamics of your environment. Imagine a workplace where everyone is well-rested: fewer mistakes, better collaboration, and a generally more positive atmosphere. Or a classroom where students retain information better and participate more actively. Enhancing cognitive function through better sleep can transform environments, making them more efficient and enjoyable for everyone involved.

Lastly, it's essential to acknowledge that sleep needs can vary from person to person. Some might feel refreshed with seven hours a night, while others need a bit more. Listening to your body and paying attention to how you feel during the day can guide you toward optimizing your sleep for better cognitive performance.

So, if you want to boost your brainpower, excel in your career, have better relationships, and make smarter decisions, prioritizing your sleep isn't an option—it's a necessity. It's time to give your brain the rest it needs to function at its absolute best.

Chapter 2:
The Biology of Sleep

Understanding the intricacies of sleep's biology is crucial for transforming your bedtime woes into restful slumber. Our bodies are governed by circadian rhythms, internal clocks synced with the Earth's 24-hour cycle, which dictate our sleep-wake patterns (Czeisler et al., 1999). These rhythms are deeply entwined with the sleep cycle, a five-stage process that repeats throughout the night. During a healthy night's sleep, you transition from light sleep to deep sleep and back, in cycles that last approximately 90 minutes (Carskadon & Dement, 2011). Each stage plays a unique role; for instance, during the Rapid Eye Movement (REM) stage, your brain becomes almost as active as it is when you're awake, facilitating essential processes like memory consolidation (Maquet, 2001). This harmonious dance between stages ensures that both the brain and body repair and rejuvenate, setting the stage for a productive day ahead. Recognizing these physiological mechanisms empowers you to respect your body's natural needs and rhythms, unlocking the potential for life-changing sleep quality.

The Sleep Cycle

At the heart of the biology of sleep beats a rhythmic dance called the sleep cycle. Understanding this cycle is crucial for anyone looking to improve their health and well-being, especially those who are sleep-deprived. The sleep cycle is composed of several distinct stages that our brains and bodies progress through multiple times each night. Grasping these stages can empower you to take control of your sleep quality, optimizing your physical and mental health.

The sleep cycle is broadly divided into two main categories: REM (rapid eye movement) sleep and non-REM sleep, each with its own unique characteristics and functions. The journey through a complete sleep cycle typically lasts about 90 to 110 minutes and repeats 4 to 6 times each night. This cycle isn't just a monotonous loop; it's a carefully orchestrated progression that our brains navigate to rejuvenate our bodies.

Non-REM sleep, which can be further divided into three stages, is where we start our trip. Stage 1 is the lightest stage of sleep. You know the feeling: drifting off, maybe dreaming for split seconds, and easily awakened by minor noises. It's a transitional phase, lasting only a few minutes as your body prepares for deeper sleep. During this stage, both the heart rate and breathing slow down, and muscle activity decreases (Carskadon & Dement, 2005).

Stage 2 is where you spend about 50% of your sleep. It's slightly deeper than stage 1, characterized by sleep spindles and K-complexes—brief bursts of brain activity that are thought to play a role in memory consolidation. During this stage, your body temperature drops and your metabolism slows down. This is your body's way of preserving energy and preparing for the more restorative stages that follow (Genzel et al., 2014).

Stage 3, also known as deep or slow-wave sleep, is the powerhouse of the sleep cycle. It's crucial for physical restoration, muscle growth, and tissue repair. Scientists believe that immune function is bolstered during this phase, with your body fighting off infections and inflammation more effectively. This stage features delta waves, which are the slowest and highest amplitude brain waves. If you've ever felt groggy and disoriented after being woken up abruptly, you were likely pulled out of this deep sleep stage (Borbély et al., 2016).

Finally, we move into REM sleep, where dreams become vivid, and our brains become almost as active as when we're awake. This stage is critically important for cognitive functions like learning and creativity. During REM sleep, your brain is sorting through information, consolidating memories, and even problem-solving. It's a mental workout, offering emotional and psychological benefits.

Interestingly, the amount of time we spend in each sleep stage isn't static throughout the night. In the first few cycles, we're bogged down more in deep non-REM sleep. However, As morning approaches, REM periods lengthen while deep sleep shortens. This nuanced architecture ensures we're hitting all required restoration checkpoints—both physically and mentally—by the time we wake up.

One of the remarkable things about the sleep cycle is its adaptability. External factors like stress, illness, or even your daily activities can alter how you cycle through these stages. For instance, if you've been sleep-deprived, your body compensates by diving more quickly into deep sleep and extending its duration. It's essentially your body catching up on "sleep debt," showing how responsive and intelligent these cycles are.

Modern challenges often disrupt these beautifully synchronized stages. Blue light from screens can delay the production of melatonin—a hormone that regulates sleep—leading to reduced REM sleep and impacting cognitive functions. High stress levels can push you to spend less time in deep sleep, weakening your immune system and making you more susceptible to illness.

What can we do to ensure our sleep cycles remain unbroken and efficient? Achieving consistency in your sleep patterns is a powerful first step. Going to bed and waking up at the same time every day—

even on weekends—helps stabilize your sleep architecture. Limiting exposure to screens at least an hour before bed can also vastly improve your cycle's effectiveness.

Moreover, understanding the uniqueness of your sleep needs can offer personalized insights. Some people might need more REM sleep to function optimally, while others may require an abundance of deep sleep. Keeping a sleep journal or using sleep-tracking tools can provide valuable data, guiding you to make more informed decisions about your sleep habits.

One often overlooked aspect is diet. Consuming foods rich in tryptophan (like turkey and milk) can promote the production of melatonin and serotonin, hormones conducive to better sleep. Equally crucial is steering clear of caffeine and alcohol close to bedtime. Caffeine can fragment your sleep cycle, and while alcohol might help you fall asleep faster, it reduces overall sleep quality by fragmenting REM sleep.

While the science behind sleep cycles is robust, it's also incredibly personal. What works for one person might not work for another, making it important to experiment and find what suits your body best. Embracing this journey leads to a healthier, more energetic version of yourself.

So, the next time you're tempted to skimp on those precious hours of shut-eye, remember: each stage of your sleep cycle has its role. Fostering a deeper understanding of these stages isn't just academic— it's practical and can be life-changing. As you begin to see sleep not as a luxury but as a non-negotiable aspect of health, you'll unlock new levels of potential in your daily life.

In summary, understanding the intricate dance of the sleep cycle can substantially impact your overall well-being. From light stages that ease you into slumber, to deep stages that repair and rejuvenate, and

REM stages that foster creativity and emotional stability—each phase is a critical performer in the symphony of your nightly rest. Respecting and optimizing this natural rhythm can pave the way for better health, greater productivity, and a more fulfilling life.

Stages of Sleep

Understanding the stages of sleep feels a bit like deciphering a fascinating but complex puzzle. Each stage has its unique characteristics and functions, all contributing to our overall sleep experience and health. And just like any great story, sleep follows a structured plot with different phases, progressing from light slumber into deeper, more restorative states, before briefly surfacing again. This cyclical progression is not only interesting but also essential to understand if we're to optimize our sleep quality.

Let's break down the stages of sleep into their main components: NREM (Non-Rapid Eye Movement) and REM (Rapid Eye Movement) sleep. These types are further divided into four sub-stages—NREM 1, NREM 2, NREM 3, and REM sleep. It's crucial to know that each of these stages plays a distinct role in our nightly rejuvenation and overall health.

NREM 1, or N1, is the lightest stage of sleep. It's that twilight zone between wakefulness and sleep where we start to drift off. Your muscles begin to relax, and you might experience hypnic jerks or sudden muscle contractions, often linked to the sensation of falling. This stage is brief, lasting only about 5-10 minutes, but it serves as the gateway to deeper sleep. During N1, your brain produces high-amplitude theta waves, and you're easily awakened (Carskadon & Dement, 2005).

Progressing into NREM 2, or N2, you move into a light sleep. This stage covers about 50% of our total sleep time. It's characterized by sleep spindles and K-complexes—sudden bursts of brain activity.

These brain oscillations are a sign that your brain is working to inhibit certain perceptions, allowing you to stay asleep and not be easily disturbed by the external environment. If you're woken up at this point, you might find yourself feeling groggy or disoriented.

The illustrious NREM 3, or N3, represents the deep sleep stage, also known as slow-wave sleep (SWS). This stage is critical for physical restoration. Think of it as the body's time to repair muscles, consolidate memories, and even bolster the immune system. N3 is characterized by delta waves—the slowest and highest-amplitude brain waves. It's much harder to wake someone from deep sleep, and if you are, you might feel incredibly disoriented. This stage usually comprises about 15-20% of total sleep time, decreasing as we age.

Finally, we plunge into REM sleep, the phase that most of us associate with vivid dreaming. Your brain activity during REM sleep is similar to that of being awake, exhibiting low-amplitude, mixed-frequency waves. What's absolutely fascinating is that although the brain is buzzing with activity, the body enters a state of temporary paralysis, preventing us from acting out our dreams—an essential safety feature, if you think about it! REM sleep is particularly vital for cognitive functions like memory consolidation, problem-solving, and emotional regulation (Stickgold, 2005).

It's vital to highlight the cyclical nature of these stages. A complete sleep cycle usually lasts about 90-110 minutes and comprises all four stages. Most people go through 4-6 cycles a night. Understanding that sleep isn't a static state but a dynamic process underscores the importance of uninterrupted sleep. Fragmenting this cycle can lead to sleep disturbances and impair the restorative functions of each stage (Carskadon & Dement, 2005).

Consider this: lack of deep NREM sleep particularly affects physical growth and recovery. If you're an athlete or physically active, this is when your body releases growth hormones (Van Cauter et al.,

2000), repairing muscles and tissues—essentially recharging your physical capabilities. Meanwhile, REM sleep lacks can detrimentally affect your cognitive abilities and emotional stability (Walker, 2009). Missing out on REM means your mind isn't processing emotions correctly, which can lead to an increase in stress, anxiety, and mood swings.

Moreover, think about the intriguing interplay between these stages and how lifestyle choices or certain disorders might influence them. Factors like stress, alcohol consumption, or sleep disorders can severely disrupt these stages, leading to decreased sleep quality and subsequent health issues. For instance, sleep apnea often impedes both REM and deep sleep stages, leaving individuals perpetually sleep-deprived despite spending enough time in bed (Peppard et al., 2000).

What's encouraging, though, is that understanding these stages empowers us to make informed choices about our sleep hygiene. By appreciating the complexity and the necessity of each sleep stage, we can prioritize habits that promote not just more sleep, but better-quality sleep. Simple changes like reducing blue light exposure before bed, maintaining a consistent sleep schedule, and engaging in regular exercise can help ensure that we glide through these stages smoothly each night.

Recognizing the stages of sleep and their respective contributions allows us to appreciate just how deliberate and structured our bodies are in maintaining overall health and well-being. Each stage is like a piece of a puzzle, and only when they all fit together perfectly can we experience the full spectrum of restorative sleep benefits.

Chapter 3:
Common Sleep Disorders

After diving into the importance and biology of sleep, it's essential to explore common sleep disorders that often upend our quest for restful nights. Insomnia, a prevalent sleep disorder, can leave you staring at the ceiling for hours, robbing you of the rejuvenation your mind and body desperately need (Roth, 2007). Meanwhile, sleep apnea—characterized by interrupted breathing—disrupts not just your sleep but also your cardiovascular health (Punjabi, 2008). Then there's Restless Leg Syndrome, forcing your legs into unrelenting motion when you should be finding peace under the sheets (Walters et al., 1996). Understanding these conditions is the first step in reclaiming your nights and, by extension, your days. The path to better sleep isn't just about knowing what's wrong but being empowered to address these issues head-on. Knowledge is your biggest ally here, helping you transform sleepless nights into ones filled with restorative, uninterrupted sleep.

Insomnia

Insomnia is one of the most prevalent sleep disorders affecting individuals today, characterized by persistent difficulty falling asleep, staying asleep, or both. This struggle leads to poor sleep quality, impacting daily functioning and overall health. It's a widespread issue, especially among professionals and students who often find themselves balancing numerous responsibilities and coping with high stress levels.

In simple terms, insomnia is both a symptom and a disorder. When it is persistent and not linked to external events like work stress or illness, it becomes known as chronic insomnia. Acute insomnia, on the other hand, is usually triggered by significant life events or environmental factors and can last days or weeks. Understanding the difference is crucial for targeting effective treatment.

Insomnia doesn't just rob people of their rest; it also steals their sense of well-being and productivity. The inability to get sufficient sleep can lead to irritability, cognitive impairments, and a diminished ability to handle everyday tasks. For those juggling demanding careers, academic work, and personal lives, consistent poor sleep can snowball into bigger issues. When insomnia lingers and becomes chronic, the impact extends far beyond mere tiredness.

Scientific research highlights that insomnia is often associated with other mental health issues, such as depression and anxiety (Baglioni et al., 2011). It becomes a vicious cycle where poor sleep exacerbates mental health issues, which in turn makes sleep even harder to come by. The long-term consequences can be severe if the cycle isn't broken.

The symptoms of insomnia can be diverse, extending beyond just sleepless nights. These might include daytime fatigue, memory issues, mood disturbances, and even a higher likelihood of making mistakes or having accidents. What's troubling is that many people with insomnia resort to unhealthy coping mechanisms like overuse of caffeine or even reliance on alcohol, which further worsen the situation.

Several factors contribute to this pervasive issue. Stress is a significant contributor to insomnia. Worrying about work deadlines, family matters, or even global events can keep your mind racing when it should be winding down. Hormonal imbalances, particularly in women, can also play a role due to the fluctuations during menstruation, pregnancy, and menopause (Katz & McHorney, 2002).

Lifestyle choices play a crucial part as well. Irregular sleep schedules, excessive screen time, and poor diet can severely disrupt your sleep patterns. It's a delicate balance, and the cumulative effect of these factors can push many into the cycle of insomnia. If you've ever lain in bed, staring at the ceiling, wondering why sleep is evading you, it's crucial to consider these contributing elements.

Treatment for insomnia varies depending on the severity and underlying causes. Cognitive Behavioral Therapy for Insomnia (CBT-I) is considered highly effective for treating chronic insomnia (Edinger et al., 2021). Unlike sleeping pills, which can lose effectiveness over time and sometimes lead to dependency, CBT-I addresses the root causes of insomnia and helps individuals to reframe negative thoughts about sleep and develop healthier sleep habits. This therapy typically involves sleep restriction, stimulus control, and learning relaxation techniques.

Pharmacological treatments can offer quick relief, but they are often best used for short-term cases of insomnia. Over-the-counter options and prescription medications can help someone get through brief periods of sleeplessness, but they are rarely a long-term solution. The focus should always be on building sustainable habits and a sleep-friendly environment.

One practical tip for managing insomnia is to establish a consistent sleep routine. Your body's internal clock, or circadian rhythm, thrives on consistency. Going to bed and waking up at the same time every day can reinforce a healthy sleep cycle. Trying pre-sleep rituals can also signal to your body that it's time to wind down. Perhaps this means reading a book, practicing relaxation exercises, or listening to calming music.

Another effective strategy involves ensuring your sleep environment is conducive to rest. A dark, cool, and quiet room can make a significant difference. Often, people overlook the basics like comfortable bedding or optimal room temperature, which can significantly enhance sleep quality. Investing in blackout curtains or white noise machines can be a game-changer for those struggling with insomnia.

For those whose insomnia is exacerbated by technology, mitigating blue light exposure is crucial. Limit screen time before bed and consider using blue light filters on devices. The aim is to minimize disruptions to your melatonin production, the hormone responsible for regulating sleep-wake cycles.

Sometimes, despite our best efforts, insomnia persists. In such cases, seeking professional help might be necessary. A sleep specialist can offer targeted solutions, ranging from advanced behavioral therapies to specialized medical interventions. Sometimes, a comprehensive review of your health can reveal underlying conditions that contribute to insomnia, such as sleep apnea or restless leg syndrome.

In conclusion, insomnia is more than just an inconvenience; it's a significant health issue that demands attention. By understanding its nature and potential treatments, you can take significant steps towards reclaiming your nights and improving overall well-being. Sustainable sleep solutions often involve a combination of behavioral changes, environmental adjustments, and sometimes professional help. Remember, good sleep isn't a luxury—it's a necessity that propels us toward achieving our best selves.

Sleep Apnea

Sleep apnea is one of the most common but underdiagnosed sleep disorders affecting millions of people worldwide. Characterized by interruptions in breathing during sleep, this condition can severely impact overall sleep quality and lead to a series of serious health problems if left untreated. Understanding sleep apnea is crucial for anyone striving to optimize their health and well-being.

There are two primary types of sleep apnea: obstructive sleep apnea (OSA) and central sleep apnea (CSA). OSA is the more common form and occurs when the muscles in the throat relax excessively, causing a temporary blockage of the airway. On the other hand, CSA happens when the brain fails to send proper signals to the muscles that control breathing. These interruptions can happen dozens or even hundreds of times per night, resulting in fragmented and non-restorative sleep.

Many people with sleep apnea are unaware they have it. Often, they're alerted to the problem by their sleep partners who notice the loud snoring or gasping for air during the night. Common symptoms include excessive daytime sleepiness, morning headaches, and difficulty concentrating. Over time, untreated sleep apnea can elevate the risk of hypertension, heart disease, stroke, and type 2 diabetes (Lavie et al., 2010).

The consequences of sleep apnea reach far beyond the individual. Sleep-deprived professionals can perform poorly at work, making errors that range from minor to catastrophic. Students with sleep apnea may find it hard to focus in class and retain information, leading to decreased academic performance. Also, the social implications are significant—imagine trying to participate in social events while battling constant fatigue.

Scientifically, the reasons why sleep apnea causes so much harm are rooted in its effects on the body's physiological functions. The repeated pauses in breathing lower blood oxygen levels, which in turn increase blood pressure and strain the cardiovascular system. This deteriorates heart health over time and can lead to arrhythmias or heart failure (Somers et al., 2008). Moreover, disrupted sleep cycles affect brain functions like memory consolidation and emotional regulation.

Diagnosing sleep apnea typically involves undergoing a sleep study, either at home or in a specialized sleep clinic. These studies monitor various indicators such as airflow, blood oxygen levels, and brain activity, providing comprehensive data that helps in diagnosing the condition accurately. Once diagnosed, treatment options vary depending on the severity of the condition and overall health of the individual.

The most well-known treatment for sleep apnea is Continuous Positive Airway Pressure (CPAP) therapy. A CPAP machine delivers a continuous stream of air through a mask worn during sleep, keeping the airway open and preventing interruptions in breathing. While many people find CPAP effective, others may struggle to adapt due to discomfort or difficulty tolerating the mask. Fortunately, there are alternative treatments available.

Oral appliances, often custom-made by dentists, can help keep the airway open by repositioning the jaw. These devices are particularly effective for those with mild to moderate obstructive sleep apnea (Sutherland et al., 2014). Surgical options also exist, ranging from minimally invasive procedures to more extensive surgeries designed to remove or shrink tissues obstructing the airway. Lifestyle changes like weight loss, quitting smoking, and avoiding alcohol before bedtime can further improve symptoms.

Let's touch on a critical aspect: the importance of individualized treatment plans. Not everyone responds to the same therapy, and it's crucial to work closely with healthcare providers to find the most effective solutions. Personalized treatment not only alleviates symptoms but also drastically reduces the risk of developing serious complications.

It's empowering to know that even small changes can make a big difference. Prioritizing nasal hygiene, for example, can enhance CPAP effectiveness. Regularly cleaning the device and ensuring a proper fit can make the experience more comfortable and increase compliance. Adhering to a consistent sleep schedule and creating an optimal sleep environment can further enhance the effectiveness of any prescribed treatment.

It's vital not to overlook the mental and emotional impact of sleep apnea. Individuals diagnosed with the disorder often feel embarrassed or frustrated, which can contribute to stress and anxiety. Support groups and counseling can offer emotional relief, allowing sufferers to share experiences and coping strategies.

Technological advancements are also paving the way for more effective and comfortable treatment options. Newer CPAP machines are quieter and more user-friendly, and innovative apps are emerging to help track sleep patterns and treatment efficacy. Research in biomedical engineering is continuously seeking ways to make sleep apnea management more accessible and less intrusive for everyone.

Public awareness campaigns play a crucial role in promoting early diagnosis and treatment. The more people know about the condition, the more likely they are to recognize the symptoms in themselves or loved ones and seek help. Thus, education is paramount, and this book aims to be part of that crucial educational effort.

In summary, sleep apnea is a prevalent and potentially serious condition that requires attention. By understanding the types, symptoms, and treatment options, you are better equipped to take control of your sleep health. Whether through medical intervention, lifestyle modifications, or support networks, effective management of sleep apnea can significantly improve quality of life. Don't let sleep apnea steal your rest—take the necessary steps to reclaim healthy and restorative sleep.

Restless Leg Syndrome

Restless Leg Syndrome (RLS) is a sleep disorder that lurks in the shadows, often going unnoticed or misdiagnosed. It's more than just an occasional leg twitch; it's a neurological condition characterized by an uncontrollable urge to move the legs, usually accompanied by uncomfortable sensations. These sensations often get worse during periods of rest or inactivity, particularly in the evening or night, making it especially problematic for achieving and maintaining good sleep. For sleep-deprived professionals, students, and anyone looking to optimize their health and well-being, understanding RLS is crucial.

Imagine lying in bed after a grueling day, looking forward to some much-needed rest, only to feel an incessant urge to move your legs. This uncontrollable need can range from mildly annoying to utterly debilitating. Symptoms typically ease with movement but return once you're still again, creating a frustrating cycle that disrupts sleep and diminishes overall quality of life. The sensations vary, described as aching, throbbing, pulling, or creeping feelings that result in continual restlessness.

The difficulty of diagnosing RLS stems from its subjective nature. Unlike disorders that can be easily observed or measured, RLS relies heavily on self-reporting. Individuals suffering from RLS often achieve relief through movement, which offers temporary relief but ultimately feeds into a cycle of disrupted sleep. This nightly battle can lead to chronic sleep deprivation, impacting work performance, cognitive function, and emotional well-being.

While the exact cause of RLS isn't entirely understood, it's believed to involve an imbalance of dopamine, a neurotransmitter responsible for sending messages to control muscle movement. According to recent studies, low levels of iron in the brain might contribute to this imbalance, as iron plays a key role in dopamine production (Allen et al., 2021). Genetics also appears to be a significant factor, with the condition often running in families.

Lifestyle choices can exacerbate the symptoms of RLS. Caffeine, alcohol, and nicotine have all been identified as potential triggers.

Reducing intake of these substances might help alleviate symptoms. Additionally, certain medications, including some antidepressants and anti-nausea drugs, can worsen RLS. Consulting with a healthcare provider about these medications is advisable if you suspect they're influencing your symptoms.

Managing RLS often requires a multifaceted approach. For starters, establishing a regular sleep routine can be incredibly beneficial. Going to bed and waking up at the same time every day helps to regulate your body's internal clock, making it easier to fall asleep and stay asleep. Relaxation techniques such as deep breathing, meditation, and gentle stretching before bed can also prepare your body for sleep and minimize the discomfort associated with RLS.

Another cornerstone in managing RLS is physical exercise, which has been shown to reduce the severity of symptoms. However, timing is key. Engaging in moderate exercise earlier in the day, rather than close to bedtime, can help mitigate symptoms without over-stimulating your body before sleep. Activities like walking, swimming, or yoga can be particularly effective.

Dietary modifications can also play a role. Since iron deficiency is linked to RLS, incorporating iron-rich foods like lean meat, beans, and leafy greens into your diet might ease symptoms. Pair these with foods high in vitamin C to enhance iron absorption. Moreover, some evidence suggests that magnesium and folate supplements may offer relief (Hening et al., 2017). However, always consult with a healthcare provider before beginning any supplementation.

When lifestyle modifications aren't enough, medical treatment is available. Dopaminergic agents, which increase dopamine levels, are commonly prescribed and can be quite effective. Other medicinal options include anticonvulsants and opioids, though these are generally considered when other treatments have failed due to their potential side effects.

Moreover, regular follow-ups with your healthcare provider are essential for managing RLS effectively. Symptom severity can fluctuate over time, requiring adjustments in treatment. Also, since RLS can be associated with other medical conditions such as peripheral neuropathy, sleep apnea, or even kidney disease, it's vital to rule out any underlying issues that could be contributing to your symptoms.

Living with RLS can be challenging, but knowing that it is a recognized medical condition can be empowering. By taking a proactive approach—whether that means lifestyle changes, seeking medical advice, or both—you can significantly improve your sleep quality and overall life satisfaction. Remember, the goal is not just temporary relief but long-term management, enabling you to reclaim those precious hours of restful sleep.

Chapter 4:
Debunking Sleep Myths

In our quest for a good night's sleep, we've all encountered well-meaning but misleading advice. Let's clear the air by debunking some common sleep myths. First, the notion that you can catch up on lost sleep over the weekend is a widespread misconception. Research shows that trying to make up for lost sleep disrupts your body's natural rhythms and worsens sleep quality over time (Van Dongen et al., 2003). Another fallacy is believing that alcohol can help you sleep better. While alcohol might make you fall asleep faster, it diminishes sleep quality by reducing REM sleep, leading to fragmentation and early awakenings (Ebrahim et al., 2013). Dispelling these myths is crucial for unlocking real, sustainable sleep improvements, so ditch the shortcuts and focus on creating lasting habits that support quality rest.

Myth 1: You Can Catch Up on Sleep Over the Weekend

It's tempting to think of sleep as a sort of bank account: rack up some sleep debt during the week, then make a "payment" with a weekend sleep-a-thon. Unfortunately, the science says otherwise. Numerous studies have shown that you can't fully compensate for poor sleep habits during the week with a couple of nights of longer sleep, no matter how appealing that may sound (Åkerstedt et al., 2009).

The most we can hope for with extra weekend sleep is a temporary reduction in sleepiness and some minor cognitive improvements.

However, these benefits are fleeting and don't erase the long-term consequences of chronic sleep deprivation, such as impaired memory, reduced cognitive function, and increased risk of chronic diseases like diabetes and heart disease (Banks et al., 2010). When we shortchange ourselves on sleep during the week, we create a cascade of detrimental effects that can't simply be undone by extra sleep over the weekend.

What's more, attempting to "catch up" on sleep by sleeping in can actually disrupt your internal body clock, or circadian rhythm, making it harder to fall asleep and wake up at appropriate times during the week. This misalignment can result in what's known as social jet lag—a state where your body clock is out of sync with your daily schedule, leading to feelings of chronic fatigue and decreased performance (Wittmann et al., 2006).

Scientific research has consistently shown the importance of maintaining a regular sleep schedule. Regular sleep patterns reinforce your body's natural circadian rhythms, helping you feel more alert and energized during the day and ensuring you get the restorative sleep you need at night (Roenneberg et al., 2012). Consistency is the cornerstone of good sleep hygiene and is far more beneficial than sporadic attempts to make up for lost sleep.

In practical terms, this means aiming to go to bed and wake up at the same time every day, even on weekends. If you're losing sleep during the week due to work, study, or social commitments, it's crucial to identify strategies to protect and prioritize your sleep. This might mean making sacrifices in other areas, but the benefits to your physical and mental health make it a worthwhile investment.

Moreover, our bodies don't loan us "extra" sleep resources to utilize later. Sleep is an immediate, restorative process that needs to happen regularly for us to function optimally. Depriving yourself of it consistently leads to cumulative deficits that impair your ability to think, react, and handle stress. Your immune system becomes compromised, making you more susceptible to illness. These deficits don't just build up; they compound, affecting every aspect of your life.

Consequently, the idea that you can "catch up" on sleep later provides a false sense of security. When you run short on sleep, your cognitive functions suffer. Your attention span shortens, your decision-making abilities weaken, and your mood sours. Sleep research shows that even one night of sleep loss can significantly affect your brain's functionality, particularly in areas like the prefrontal cortex, which governs complex thought and decision-making (Walker, 2017).

So, what should you do if you find yourself constantly tired, even with those weekend sleep marathons? Start by evaluating your daily habits and evening routines. Are you staying up late binge-watching shows or scrolling through social media? Are you consuming caffeine too late in the day? Identify the behaviors that may be cutting into your sleep and work on modifying them.

Creating a wind-down ritual can also be beneficial. Establishing a routine that signals to your body it's time to prepare for sleep can make a significant difference. This could include activities like reading, taking a warm bath, or practicing relaxation techniques. The goal is to create a peaceful environment that encourages your body to transition into sleep mode.

Also, the quality of sleep matters as much as quantity. High-quality, uninterrupted sleep does more for restoring your body and mind than an equal amount of fitful or fragmented sleep. Addressing issues that impact sleep quality, such as noise, light, and temperature, can help you get the most out of your sleeping hours and reduce the temptation to "catch up" later.

In conclusion, the myth that you can catch up on sleep over the weekend does more harm than good. It misleadingly suggests that it's okay to accumulate sleep debt, which can have a profound and negative impact on your health. The most effective way to reap the benefits of sleep is through consistency—prioritizing a steady sleep schedule each night, rather than relying on weekend compensation.

Prioritizing your sleep means valuing those consistent daily habits. While the occasional late night might be unavoidable, making a habit out of them isn't sustainable. Create a sleep schedule that honors your need for rest. Aim to get between 7 to 9 hours of sleep each night, and don't let the allure of the weekend sleep-in fool you into thinking it's a viable solution.

Ultimately, don't shortchange yourself by thinking you can make it all up later; your body and mind need regular, consistent sleep. Make it a non-negotiable part of your routine, and you'll find yourself healthier, happier, and far more productive.

Myth 2: Alcohol Helps You Sleep

It's a myth as old as time, but let's cut to the chase: Alcohol does not help you sleep well. Sure, you might feel drowsy after a couple of glasses of wine, but the story doesn't end there. In reality, alcohol is a sneaky disruptor that causes more harm than good when it comes to achieving a restful night's sleep.

While it's true that alcohol can make you fall asleep faster, it wreaks havoc on the quality of your sleep. Studies have shown that alcohol affects your sleep cycle, particularly the REM (Rapid Eye Movement) stage, which is crucial for cognitive functions like memory consoledation and mood regulation (Ebrahim et al., 2013). When you drink, your body spends less time in REM sleep, leading to fragmented sleep patterns. You might find yourself waking up multiple times during the night without even realizing it.

So, why do so many people believe that alcohol helps them sleep? The answer lies in the initial sedative effect of alcohol. It acts on the central nervous system, slowing down brain function and relaxing your muscles (Roehrs & Roth, 2001). This can make you feel drowsy and lead to that initial drift into slumber more quickly. However, the problem arises later in the night, when the body starts to metabolize the alcohol. As the sedative effects wear off, a rebound effect kicks in, causing increased arousal and sleep fragmentation.

Let's also not forget that alcohol can significantly exacerbate sleep disorders like sleep apnea. Alcohol relaxes the muscles in your throat, increasing the likelihood of airway obstruction and causing snoring or even pauses in breathing. This is especially troubling for individuals who already suffer from sleep apnea, as alcohol can make their symptoms markedly worse (Mason et al., 2015).

You might be thinking, "But I've had nights where a drink helped me sleep just fine!" Remember, it's not just about falling asleep; it's about the quality of that sleep. If you're waking up feeling groggy, unrefreshed, or more tired than when you went to bed, alcohol could be the culprit. The sleep disruptions caused by alcohol are subtle but accumulate over time, resulting in a significant sleep debt that affects your overall health and well-being.

We can't stress enough how important high-quality sleep is for optimal cognitive function and overall health. Alcohol-induced sleep might feel deeper, but it's far from restorative. It's like filling up your gas tank with low-quality fuel – you'll drive, but your engine will eventually suffer. When you swap alcohol-induced drowsiness for actual, unmedicated sleep, you'll experience fewer middle-of-the-night awakenings and spend more time in the rejuvenating deep and REM stages of sleep.

If you're someone who enjoys a nightly drink, consider reducing consumption gradually. You don't have to go cold turkey. Start by swapping out the last drink of the night for non-alcoholic options like herbal teas, which can have their own sleep-inducing properties.

Chamomile tea, for example, has mild sedative effects that could naturally help you wind down without disturbing your sleep architecture.

Still, social rituals involving alcohol are deeply ingrained in our culture. Whether it's a glass of wine with dinner or cocktails with friends, abstaining entirely might feel isolating or overly restrictive. However, moderation is key. Studies suggest that consuming alcohol at least four to six hours before bedtime minimizes its detrimental effects on sleep (Roehrs & Roth, 2001). Planning your last drink for earlier in the evening allows your body enough time to metabolize the alcohol before sleep.

Moreover, adopting better pre-sleep routines can make it easier to replace that drink. Develop calming habits that signal to your body it's time to wind down. Techniques such as deep breathing, light stretching, or even reading a book can shift your focus away from the need for a nightcap. Eventually, these activities can become triggers for relaxation and sleep, offering a healthier pathway to rest.

In conclusion, while the occasional drink won't spell disaster for your sleep patterns, making it a nightly habit can severely compromise the quality of your sleep. Alcohol might seem like a quick fix to fall asleep, but it's a false friend that does more harm than good. Armed with better knowledge, you can make choices that genuinely support restful, restorative sleep. For those who are serious about improving their sleep quality, the understanding that alcohol disrupts sleep is a vital step toward more energized and productive days.

Chapter 5:
Creating the Perfect
Sleep Environment

A restful night's sleep is not just about the hours you log but also about the quality of your sleep environment. Imagine your bedroom as a sanctuary—the ultimate retreat from the chaos of daily life. A key player in this setup is eliminating clutter, allowing your brain to associate the space strictly with relaxation and sleep (Stutz et al., 2019). Dimming the lights and keeping the room cool—somewhere between 60-67 degrees Fahrenheit—can signal to your body that it's time to wind down, optimizing both the duration and quality of your sleep (Murphy & Campbell, 1997). It's also essential to invest in a good mattress and pillows that support your spine and cushion your joints, thereby preventing any midnight tosses and turns that might disrupt your slumber (Jacobson et al., 2010). Blackout curtains can help mitigate the negative impact of artificial light and natural disruptions, promoting a darker, more restful environment. These seemingly small adjustments can make a monumental difference in how you feel when you wake up, ultimately empowering you to achieve a state of well-being and peak productivity. So, let's take tangible steps to transform your bedroom into a sleep-friendly oasis and elevate your nightly rest to optimal levels.

Bedroom Setup

Your bedroom should be a sanctuary dedicated to slumber. This is non-negotiable if you want to optimize your sleep quality. It all starts with creating an environment that signals to your brain that it's time to wind down and rest. Studies have shown that the design and setup of your bedroom can make a significant impact on how well you sleep (Gong et al., 2016).

First off, let's talk about the bed itself. Your bed is the throne of your sleep kingdom and choosing the right mattress and pillow can change your life—seriously. A mattress that's either too firm or too soft can lead to discomfort, and hence, compromised sleep quality. Similarly, pillows with the right ergonomic support are essential for maintaining proper neck alignment throughout the night (Jacobson et al., 2010). When testing out mattresses, lay on them in the store for at least ten minutes to gauge comfort. Don't rush this decision.

Beyond comfort, consider the size of your bed. If you're frequently tossing and turning or share your bed with a partner, upgrading to a larger mattress may alleviate some of that discomfort. Think about it: more space means fewer disturbances from your partner's movements, and consequently, a more restful night.

Then, there's the matter of your bed linens. We often overlook this, but the type of sheets, blankets, and covers you use can affect your sleep temperature regulation and overall comfort. Opt for fabrics that are breathable like cotton or linen to help maintain a comfortable body temperature throughout the night. Also, keep your linens clean. Dust mites and allergens can accumulate in your bedding and contribute to sleep issues (Arlian et al., 2001).

Another underrated aspect is the layout of the bedroom itself. Clutter can be a physical manifestation of stress, and sleeping in a cluttered environment can actually make it harder to fall asleep. Just think about how you feel when you walk into a messy room versus a tidy one. Invest some time in keeping your bedroom organized. Put away laundry, clear off the nightstand, and always make your bed. These small acts can make the space feel more inviting and restful.

But what about the colors and décor? Believe it or not, the colors you choose can either calm or energize you. Soft blues, greens, and earthy tones have a calming effect and are generally recommended for bedrooms (Burkley et al., 2020). On the other hand, bright and bold colors can be stimulating, which is precisely what you don't want when you're trying to sleep.

It's also worth mentioning scents. Aromatherapy has gained traction as an effective way to improve sleep quality. Essential oils such as lavender have been scientifically proven to have a calming effect that can aid in falling asleep faster and achieving a more restful sleep (Hwang & Shin, 2015). Consider using a diffuser with essential oils or a pillow spray to incorporate this into your nightly routine.

Let's not forget about noise levels. Your bedroom should be as quiet as possible. Noise pollution can disrupt your sleep cycle, leading to fragmented sleep and a restless night. Soundproofing your room can be achieved by using thick curtains, carpets, or noise-cancelling machines. If absolute silence is unsettling, consider a white noise machine or a fan to create a consistent, soothing background noise.

Lighting also plays a crucial role. During the night, your room should be dark—ideally pitch black. This is because our bodies are hardwired to sleep when it's dark. Use blackout curtains to keep outside light from seeping into your room. If you need some light, such as a night light, make sure it's dim and has a red or orange hue. Blue and white lights can trick your brain into thinking it's daytime, suppressing melatonin production and keeping you awake (Cajochen et al., 2011).

However, don't underestimate the importance of natural light in the morning. Exposure to natural light when you wake up can help regulate your circadian rhythm, making it easier for you to fall asleep and wake up at consistent times. Position your bed to take advantage of morning sunlight or consider using a sunrise alarm clock to simulate this effect.

Another pro tip? Don't let technology invade your sleep sanctuary. Laptops, smartphones, and even televisions can be major distractions and sources of blue light. One study published in the journal "Sleep Health" found that the presence of these devices in the bedroom was associated with poorer sleep quality and reduced sleep duration (Shochat et al., 2019). Make it a rule: no screens in the bedroom.

This brings us to the temperature of your room. A cool room, around 60-67 degrees Fahrenheit, is optimal for sleep. Your body's core temperature naturally dips when you sleep, and a cooler environment can assist in that process. Consider investing in a programmable thermostat so that your room is always at the perfect temperature when it's time for bed. If you live in a colder climate, layering your bedding can help you adjust your comfort levels more precisely.

In summary, setting up your bedroom for optimal sleep involves a comprehensive approach: from choosing the right bed and linens to managing light, noise, and temperature. It might seem like a lot to consider, but remember, these adjustments are small changes that collectively make a significant impact. Investing time and effort in creating the perfect sleep environment is one of the most actionable steps you can take to improve your health and well-being. Here's to better sleep and brighter days ahead!

Temperature and Lighting

When considering the perfect sleep environment, temperature and lighting are two critical variables that can substantially affect the quality of your sleep. Let's delve deeper into how managing these elements can optimize your slumber.

To start with, let's talk about temperature. Ever noticed how it's easier to fall asleep in a slightly cooler room? This isn't just a coincidence. Scientific research confirms people generally sleep better in cooler environments. The ideal room temperature for most people lies between 60-67 degrees Fahrenheit (NINDS, 2018). When your body gets ready to sleep, your core temperature decreases slightly. This process facilitates the transition from wakefulness to sleep and helps maintain sleep throughout the night.

Maintaining an optimal bedroom temperature can work wonders for those who struggle with sleep quality. Being too hot or too cold can disrupt your sleep stages, specifically the Rapid Eye Movement (REM) sleep where most dreaming occurs and which is essential for emotional and cognitive restoration.

Managing your home's heating, ventilation, and air conditioning (HVAC) systems to maintain a stable temperature at night might be worth the investment. Additionally, consider the benefits of breathable bedding materials like cotton or linen, which can help regulate body temperature more effectively than synthetics. In winter, a good strategy is to layer your bedding. This allows you to adjust to your comfort level easily, enhancing both warmth and breathability.

Next up, lighting. Exposure to light and darkness significantly influences our sleep-wake cycles, commonly known as circadian rhythms (Gooley et al., 2011). During the day, light exposure keeps us awake and alert, while darkness signals the body that it's time to wind down. This is primarily due to the production of melatonin, a hormone that gets inhibited by light and facilitates sleep in darkness.

A well-lit environment during the day is crucial, especially for those whose jobs or studies keep them indoors. Natural light is the best, but if you're in an environment lacking daylight, consider investing in a high-quality light therapy lamp. Aim for at least 30 minutes of exposure to simulate natural daylight conditions.

As the evening rolls around, your goal should be reducing light exposure. Dim the lights around your home a few hours before bedtime. Using blackout curtains can help prevent ambient light from disturbing your sleep. Additionally, opting for red or amber reading lights instead of blue or white lights can be less disruptive to melatonin production (Cajochen et al., 2011).

Modern life comes with its share of challenges, one of which is our addiction to screens. Phones, tablets, and computers emit blue light, which is known to mess with our circadian rhythms. While we'll get into the details of managing screen time later, it's worth noting here that reducing screen exposure an hour or two before bed can immensely improve sleep quality.

Creating a relaxing pre-sleep atmosphere plays a role in conditioning your body for rest. Warm, dim lighting induces a calming effect, signaling your body to start producing melatonin. Lighting a couple of candles or using a low-wattage lamp can set the perfect tone for winding down.

Sometimes, achieving the ideal sleep environment involves making minor adjustments to your living space. Think about using temperature-regulating gadgets, such as a smart thermostat or a bedroom fan, to maintain that sweet spot between 60-67 degrees. For lighting, dimmer switches and smart bulbs can offer the versatility to create a restful environment that aligns with your sleep schedule.

In essence, investing in creating the right balance of temperature and lighting in your bedroom isn't just about comfort. It's a scientifically-backed approach to improve sleep quality, which in turn can have a positive impact on your overall health, cognitive functions, and quality of life.

We often underestimate the power of a well-engineered sleeping environment. Adjusting your room temperature and dimming the lights can offer an almost immediate improvement in your ability to fall and stay asleep. And remember: good sleep is one of the best investments you can make in your well-being.

Chapter 6:
The Role of Nutrition in Sleep

How many times have you heard that you are what you eat? Let's take it up a notch: you are how you sleep, and the two are intricately linked. Nutrition plays a pivotal role in determining the quality of your sleep, and finally understanding this connection can be a game-changer in your quest for restorative rest. From the time we sip our morning coffee to that midnight craving for a snack, the foods we consume can either be our allies or adversaries in the pursuit of good sleep. For instance, consuming foods rich in tryptophan, like turkey and dairy, can boost serotonin levels, consequently improving sleep quality (Bravo et al., 2013). On the flip side, foods high in sugar or caffeine can be disruptive, interfering with your ability to fall and stay asleep (Sivertsen et al., 2010). Imagine using your plate as a toolkit to engineer better sleep! By choosing nutrient-dense foods and maintaining balanced meals throughout the day, you're setting the stage for a smoother transition into slumber. It's not just about what you eat, but also when you eat. Understanding the rhythm of nutrient intake can help you synchronize your body's internal clock, enhancing both sleep latency and duration (Peuhkuri et al., 2012). So, let's invest in our nightly recharge not just by creating the perfect sleep environment or cutting down on screen time, but also by making our diet work for us, one meal at a time.

Foods That Promote Sleep

Getting a good night's sleep doesn't start when your head hits the pillow. It begins with what you put on your plate hours beforehand. Nutrition can significantly affect the quality of your sleep. So, let's talk about foods that can set you up for this essential nightly rejuvenation.

You might be surprised to learn that certain foods are natural sleep promoters. The amino acid tryptophan, for instance, is a precursor to serotonin, a neurotransmitter that helps regulate mood and sleep. Because serotonin is also converted into melatonin, the hormone that signals your body it's time to wind down, incorporating tryptophan-rich foods into your diet can help improve sleep quality.

Ever wondered why Thanksgiving dinner makes you feel sleepy? Turkey is rich in tryptophan, and it's often accompanied by carbohydrate-rich sides like mashed potatoes, which can further boost serotonin levels. Similarly, other tryptophan-rich foods include chicken, fish, nuts, seeds, tofu, and dairy products (Fernstrom, 2016).

Dark leafy greens like spinach and kale are high in magnesium—a mineral known for its calming effects. Magnesium helps activate the parasympathetic nervous system, which is responsible for making you feel relaxed and calm. In fact, studies have found that magnesium deficiency is linked to difficulty falling and staying asleep (Wienecke et al., 2016). So, a well-tossed salad might be more than a health choice; it's a sleep investment.

Don't underestimate the power of carbohydrates. Complex carbohydrates such as whole grains, sweet potatoes, and brown rice have a sleep-enhancing impact. They help increase the availability of tryptophan in the brain. This is particularly helpful when you consume them in the evening, creating a natural synergy with other sleep-friendly foods.

Herbal teas like chamomile and valerian root have been used for centuries as sleep remedies. Chamomile tea contains the antioxidant apigenin, which binds to certain receptors in your brain that may decrease anxiety and initiate sleep (Zheng et al., 2017). Valerian root is often used as a herbal remedy for insomnia and has been shown to help people fall asleep faster and improve sleep quality.

Bananas are another food item that can help ease you into sleep. They're rich in magnesium and potassium, both of which are natural muscle relaxants. Plus, they have vitamin B6, which is necessary for the conversion of tryptophan to serotonin.

Ever thought about adding some fish to your evening meals? Fatty fish like salmon, mackerel, and tuna are high in omega-3 fatty acids and vitamin D, which both play roles in serotonin regulation. Research suggests that a higher intake of omega-3 can improve sleep quality (Garfinkel et al., 1997). So not only are you protecting your heart, but you're also potentially helping your sleep.

Cherry juice, specifically tart cherry juice, has been studied for its ability to improve sleep quality. Cherries are a natural source of melatonin and drinking tart cherry juice has been linked to longer and more refreshing sleep (Pigeon et al., 2010). It's a simple, natural, and tasty way to boost your melatonin levels.

Almonds and walnuts are not just nutritional powerhouses for general health; they also contribute to better sleep. Almonds provide an excellent source of magnesium, while walnuts contain melatonin and healthy fats that help to maintain sleep patterns.

Timing is everything when it comes to eating for sleep. Try to consume these foods about two to three hours before bedtime. Eating too close to bedtime can cause discomfort and indigestion, which can keep you awake.

Let's talk about dairy for a moment. Warm milk is often cited as a traditional sleep aid. It's not just an old wives' tale—milk contains tryptophan and has a soothing effect that can help ease you into sleep. Plus, the calcium in dairy products helps the brain use tryptophan to manufacture melatonin.

Whole grains such as oatmeal provide more than just morning nourishment. Oats are rich in melatonin and complex carbohydrates that can help you fall asleep faster. The granola bar you enjoy in the morning might just become your evening wind-down snack.

Certain fruits are also exceptionally good at promoting sleep. Kiwifruit, for instance, has been shown to significantly improve sleep onset, duration, and efficiency (Lin et al., 2011). This green marvel is packed with a variety of sleep-promoting compounds, including antioxidants and serotonin.

In your pursuit of quality rest, it might also help to consider seeds like pumpkin seeds and flaxseeds. Pumpkin seeds are a convenient source of tryptophan, while flaxseeds provide omega-3 fatty acids, which have been shown to help people fall asleep faster and improve sleep quality.

The humble avocado, packed with healthy fats and magnesium, can also make a beneficial addition to your pre-sleep diet. These nutrients promote the production of sleep-inducing hormones and provide a sense of calm.

So there you have it: the edible arsenal for a better night's sleep. When chosen carefully, your meals can be the best sleep aid ever. Lifestyle changes, including dietary adjustments, don't have to be daunting. In fact, making such modifications can be relatively simple and deliciously rewarding.

Incorporating these foods into your daily routine is not about drastic changes; it's about making sleep-friendly choices consistently.

You don't need a complete overhaul of your diet. Instead, add in a handful of nuts here, a piece of fatty fish there, or a bedtime glass of tart cherry juice. Small changes can lead to significant improvements.

Remember, better sleep is often about the little choices you make each day. Let your diet be an ally in your quest for rest. Eating for optimal sleep is not just possible; it's practical and enjoyable. By doing so, you're setting the stage for a more restful, restorative, and ultimately more joyful life.

Foods to Avoid Before Bed

We all want a good night's sleep, but sometimes even our best efforts aren't enough. What many of us might not realize is that what we eat—especially close to bedtime—can seriously impact how well we sleep. It's not just about quantity but quality, too. So, let's dive into the foods you should definitely avoid before hitting the sack to ensure you get that rejuvenating sleep you crave.

First on the list is *caffeine*. We all know that coffee can keep us awake, but caffeine isn't just hiding in your cup of joe. It's also in certain teas, chocolate, some pain relievers, and even ice cream. Caffeine blocks adenosine, a chemical that makes you feel sleepy, and increases adrenaline production (Smith, 2002). To minimize its disruptive effects, try to cut off your caffeine intake at least six hours before bedtime.

Spicy foods and heavy meals should also be avoided. They can cause heartburn, indigestion, and general discomfort—none of which are conducive to a restful night. Chile peppers and other spicy ingredients can actually elevate your body temperature, making it harder for you to fall asleep (Habeeb & Gellai, 2020). Instead, consider lighter, milder alternatives if you need a late-night snack.

Sugary and high-carb foods are another category to watch. Eating cookies, cakes, or even large portions of pasta or bread before bed can spike your blood sugar levels. High insulin levels can disturb your sleep cycle and make you wake up in the middle of the night (Glynn, 2015). If you do crave something sweet, a small piece of fruit or a handful of nuts is a much better option.

You've probably heard that you shouldn't drink too much *water* before bed, and that's for a good reason. Consuming large amounts of any liquid can lead to frequent bathroom trips throughout the night, which can be highly disruptive. Aim to get your hydration during the day and limit fluid intake during the last hour or two before bed.

Alcohol can be a tricky one. While a nightcap might make you feel drowsy initially, alcohol affects your sleep stages, particularly the REM cycle, leading to fragmented sleep (Roehrs & Roth, 2001). The result? You wake up feeling groggy rather than refreshed. It's best to avoid alcohol at least a few hours before bedtime.

Moreover, dairy products, particularly high-fat varieties like cheese and ice cream, should be taken with caution. These foods can cause digestive issues like indigestion or even more severe discomfort such as acid reflux, disrupting your sleep process (Fass, 2005).

Fast food and other *processed foods* are also not your friends when it comes to sleep. They often contain high amounts of sodium and preservatives, which can lead to bloating and discomfort. More surprisingly, some processed foods contain hidden sugars and caffeine, further impacting your ability to fall asleep (Eckel et al., 2014).

You've got to be aware of *citrus fruits* as well. While packed with vitamin C, they can be highly acidic, causing stomach discomfort or heartburn for some people. It would be better to have these energizing fruits earlier in the day rather than at bedtime.

If you're tempted by a midnight snack or a late dinner, opt for foods that support rather than sabotage your sleep. Try small amounts of foods rich in tryptophan, magnesium, and melatonin, such as turkey, bananas, or a handful of almonds. These can actually prepare your body for sleep.

Finally, we have to talk about *large meals*. Eating a big feast late at night can be a sure-fire way to ensure you're tossing and turning in discomfort. When you consume large amounts of food, your body works hard to digest it, which can make falling asleep difficult. Aim for balanced, moderate meals in the evening and keep late-night snacking to a minimum.

Let's be real: life happens, and sometimes you might find yourself hungry late at night. Just keep these guidelines in mind, and you'll be well on your way to better sleep. Eating smarter, especially as the day winds down, can make a world of difference in how refreshed you feel in the morning.

Chapter 7:
The Impact of Technology
on Sleep

In our hyper-connected world, technology's omnipresence has a profound impact on our sleep quality, often more detrimental than we realize. The pervasive use of smartphones, tablets, and laptops disrupts our circadian rhythm through blue light exposure, effectively tricking our brains into thinking it's still daylight and thereby delaying melatonin production (Chang et al., 2015). This isn't just about screen time before bed; it's also about how constant notifications and the very nature of digital interactions can keep our minds in a state of heightened alertness long after we've powered down for the night (Cain & Gradisar, 2010). Managing screen time is crucial, and involves practical strategies like utilizing blue light filters, setting screen curfews, and creating tech-free zones in your home. This chapter dives into how small, actionable changes can safeguard our sleep, while keeping us connected in a balanced way.

Blue Light Exposure

Ever noticed how staring at your phone or laptop late at night seems to make falling asleep so much harder? You're not alone. One of the most significant impacts technology has on our sleep lies in the blue light emitted by our screens. Whether it's the smartphone you're scrolling through in bed or the laptop you're working on late into the night, these devices can seriously mess with your sleep.

Blue light is a part of the visible light spectrum, which also includes red, orange, yellow, green, and violet light. Blue light has the shortest wavelength and the highest energy, making it particularly influential on our body's physiological processes, specifically our sleep-wake cycle, also known as the circadian rhythm. Our eyes' retinas contain photoreceptor cells that are particularly sensitive to blue light, which directly influences the production of melatonin, the hormone that regulates sleep.

Think of the circadian rhythm as your body's natural clock. It regulates not just sleep, but a variety of bodily functions, from hormone release to body temperature. When the sun sets, the brain ramps up the production of melatonin, signaling it's time to wind down and prepare for sleep. However, exposure to blue light, especially during the evening hours, can suppress melatonin production, deceiving your brain into thinking it's still daytime (Chang et al., 2015). This repression of melatonin delays the onset of sleep and makes it harder for you to fall asleep when you finally do hit the bed.

In our modern world, it's almost impossible to escape screens. Be it for work, leisure, or essential communication, screens dominate our daily interactions. Thus, it becomes crucial to manage blue light exposure wisely. Cutting down on screen time before bed can mitigate the adverse effects on sleep. Ideally, experts recommend shutting off devices at least an hour before bedtime to allow melatonin levels to rise naturally (Czeisler, 2013). Yet, the practicality of this advice can be challenging given our fast-paced lives.

Software solutions like Night Shift on iOS or f.lux for computers can help reduce the amount of blue light emitted by screens, making them emit warmer tones in the evening (Lockley et al., 2017). These adjustments can lessen the impact on melatonin suppression, although they aren't a magical cure. The best course of action remains clear: the less screen time before bed, the better.

Interestingly, the problem goes beyond just hindering the ability to fall asleep. Prolonged blue light exposure also affects the quality of your sleep. Research indicates that individuals who use electronic devices before bed tend to get less REM sleep, the stage of sleep crucial for cognitive functions like memory consolidation and emotional regulation (Wood et al., 2013). Reduced REM sleep can lead to waking up feeling groggy, reducing overall productivity and well-being.

For those sleep-deprived professionals and students constantly grappling with deadlines, sleep quality becomes paramount. Interrupted or shallow sleep can lead to cognitive decline, mood disturbances, and diminished performance. Therefore, understanding and mitigating blue light exposure becomes not just a luxury but a necessity for optimizing sleep and, consequently, overall health.

Even the brightness of artificial indoor lighting can mislead your brain. Many of us underestimate the impact of the environment we spend our evenings in. Traditional incandescent bulbs tend to emit less blue light compared to the modern LED lights that have become popular. Opt for dim, warm lighting in the evenings to help signal your brain that it's time to prepare for sleep.

Studies also suggest that it's not just the presence of blue light, but also the duration and timing of exposure that matter. A brief glance at your phone might not be as detrimental as scrolling through social media for an hour before bed. The latter prolongs the exposure, giving your brain sustained signals that it's still daytime.

Blue light exposure's impacts aren't limited to our own bedrooms. Think about shift workers who are up at odd hours and constantly exposed to bright lights—both artificial and blue light from screens. For such individuals, maintaining a regular sleep schedule is already challenging. Adding blue light into the mix can exacerbate the difficulty in achieving restful sleep, further stressing the importance of controlling light exposure.

It's also important to recognize that not all blue light is bad. During the daytime, exposure to natural blue light from the sun helps keep us awake, alert, and significantly improves mood. What's problematic is the misalignment of blue light exposure with our natural circadian rhythms, leading to sleep issues. This misalignment is part of why so many sleep-deprived professionals and students find themselves in a vicious cycle—struggling with productivity by day and sleep by night.

So, what's the actionable takeaway here? Start by incorporating healthier screen habits. Consider setting an alarm or reminder on your phone to alert you when it's time to shut down for the evening. Introduce habits like reading a physical book, practicing relaxation techniques, or engaging in low-light, screen-free activities as part of your bedtime routine. Small, consistent changes can pave the way for more significant improvements in sleep quality.

In conclusion, the ubiquitous blue light emitted by our screens plays a disruptive role in our sleep quality and overall well-being. By under-standing its impact and taking steps to mitigate its effects, we can aim for a more rested and rejuvenated state. Technology isn't going anywhere, but how we interact with it, especially during the evening, can significantly determine the quality of our precious sleep.

Managing Screen Time

Modern technology has revolutionized our daily lives, offering incredible conveniences but also posing significant challenges when it comes to our sleep. For many, screens have become an integral part of daily existence, whether for work, entertainment, or staying connected. But managing screen time is crucial for fostering better sleep quality.

As we're about to explore, it's not just the presence of screens but how, when, and where we use them that makes all the difference.

We've all been there: scrolling through social media or binge-watching TV shows late into the night. The allure of digital content is potent and hard to resist, especially after a long, stressful day. But what does this do to our sleep? As it turns out, quite a lot. The issue with screen time, particularly before bed, is twofold. First, screens emit blue light, which interferes with our natural sleep-wake cycles. Second, engaging with content, whether work-related or purely for entertainment, can keep our minds engaged and alert at times when we should be winding down.

Blue light exposure is perhaps one of the most well-documented culprits in sleep disruption. This type of light affects the production of the sleep hormone melatonin, delaying its release and making it harder for us to fall asleep (Cajochen et al., 2006). The light emitted by screens on our phones, tablets, and computers mimics daylight, which tricks our brains into thinking it's still daytime. Consequently, our internal clocks, or circadian rhythms, are thrown off, leading to delayed sleep onset.

Beyond the basic biology of light exposure, there are also psychological aspects to consider. When we're consuming content—especially interactive or emotionally stimulating content—it keeps our brains in a heightened state of alertness. This is the opposite of what we need for restful sleep. Studies have shown that engaging in stimulating activities on screens can increase stress and anxiety levels, further complicating our ability to relax and drift into slumber (Hale & Guan, 2015).

So what can we do? The first step in managing screen time is setting clear boundaries. Designate specific times when you'll unplug, especially in the hours leading up to bedtime. Creating a digital curfew helps sever the ties between screen time and rest time. Ideally, you should aim to power down all electronic devices at least an hour before bed. If this sounds like a tall order, start small: even reducing screen time by 30 minutes before sleep can have a noticeable impact.

In instances where you need to use screens in the evening, technology offers some solutions. Many devices now come with blue light filters or "night modes"—features designed to reduce blue light exposure. These can be beneficial but keep in mind that while they reduce blue light, they don't eliminate the issue entirely. If you still need some screen time, consider wearing blue light-blocking glasses as an extra layer of protection.

Another crucial aspect of managing screen time is focusing on the type of content you consume. Aim for calming and relaxing material if you absolutely must use screens before bed. Reading a book on an e-reader with a backlit screen set to warmer tones is a better option than checking emails or watching an action-packed movie. The goal is to reduce emotional and mental stimulation.

Moreover, establishing a pre-sleep routine that involves activities away from screens can work wonders. Reading a physical book, taking a warm bath, or practicing relaxation techniques like deep breathing or light stretching can signal to your body that it's time to wind down. Mindfulness and meditation are also excellent alternatives, helping you shift focus from the digital world to your internal world (Hülsheger et al., 2015).

It's also worth rethinking where you use screens. Make your bedroom a tech-free zone. Reserve this space for rest and relaxation to create a strong mental association between your bed and sleep. When you use your bed as an office or entertainment center, it blurs the lines, making it harder for your mind to shut down when it's time to sleep.

Given the ubiquitous nature of screens in our lives, it's nearly impossible to cut them out completely. Instead, the focus should be on mindful use. Keep an eye on your overall screen time, not just before bed but throughout the day. Long hours in front of a screen can lead to what's often referred to as "screen fatigue," characterized by eye strain, headaches, and, of course, sleep disruptions. Balancing screen time with activities that don't involve screens—like talking a walk, socializing face-to-face, or engaging in hobbies—can benefit your overall well-being and, by extension, your sleep.

Awareness is the first step toward effective screen time management. Tracking how much time you spend on various devices can provide valuable insights. Most smartphones now come with built-in tools for monitoring screen time, breaking it down by apps and usage types. Use these tools to identify patterns and make targeted adjustments. Maybe you're losing an hour to social media every night without realizing it. Or perhaps work emails are stretching into your evening routine, creating a cycle of stress and sleep disruption. Seeing the cold, hard data can be the wake-up call you need to make meaningful changes.

In conclusion, managing screen time is critically important for improving sleep quality. It's a multi-faceted approach requiring both practical strategies and a shift in mindset. By setting boundaries, using helpful tools, and creating a screen-free pre-sleep routine, you can mitigate the negative impacts of screen time. Balancing technology use with other activities and being mindful of how and when you use screens can pave the way for more restful, rejuvenating sleep. Remember, it's not about completely eliminating screens but using them wisely to support your health and well-being.

Chapter 8:
Stress and Sleep

Stress and sleep share an intricate, often tumultuous relationship. Elevated stress levels can disrupt our sleep patterns, leading to a vicious cycle where lack of sleep further exacerbates stress, harming both mental and physical health (Gunnar & Quevedo, 2007). When we are stressed, our body's sympathetic nervous system remains activated, leading to cortisol spikes that wreak havoc on our ability to achieve quality sleep (Buckley & Schatzberg, 2005). We need to find effective strategies to mitigate stress—whether it is through relaxation techniques, mindfulness, or meditation—to nurture better sleep hygiene. Research demonstrates that mindfulness practices not only lessen stress but also enhance overall sleep quality, paving the way for more restorative and uninterrupted slumber (Winbush et al., 2007). By prioritizing stress management and integrating calming practices into our daily routine, we can unlock the door to a healthier, more fulfilling life, free from the relentless grip of sleepless nights and daytime grogginess.

Relaxation Techniques

In a world brimming with endless emails, demanding deadlines, and constant notifications, finding effective relaxation techniques can be the bridge to a peaceful night's sleep. Stress is a natural part of life, but it's how we manage it that can make or break our sleep quality. Let's dive into some scientifically-backed methods you can easily integrate into your daily routine to melt away stress and invite restful slumber.

First and foremost, deep breathing exercises can make a significant difference. When you engage in deep breathing, it activates the body's parasympathetic nervous system, which is responsible for rest and digestion. This can help to counteract the effects of stress, reducing cortisol levels and making it easier to fall asleep. An easy way to get started is the 4-7-8 technique: inhale through your nose for 4 seconds, hold your breath for 7 seconds, and then exhale through your mouth for 8 seconds. Repeat this cycle several times, and you'll likely feel your body start to relax (Harvard Health, 2020).

Listening to calming music can also be a highly effective way to unwind before bed. Music has an uncanny ability to influence our emotions and physical state. Studies have shown that listening to soothing tunes can lower blood pressure, slow your pulse, and reduce levels of stress hormones. Opt for genres like classical music, jazz, or ambient soundscapes. You might even create a bedtime playlist that's tailored to soothe your nerves and lull you into a peaceful state.

Progressive muscle relaxation (PMR) is another powerful tool in your relaxation arsenal. Developed by Dr. Edmund Jacobson in the 1920s, PMR involves tensing and then slowly relaxing different muscle groups in your body. This technique can help reduce stress and anxiety, which are common culprits in sleep disturbances. Start from your toes and work your way up to your head, clenching each muscle group for a few seconds before releasing. By the end of the exercise, you should feel a noticeable drop in physical tension, making it easier to drift off to sleep (Hargrove, 2019).

Aromatherapy, the use of essential oils for therapeutic benefits, has been gaining traction as a relaxation technique. Lavender, in particular, has been studied extensively for its calming properties. A few drops of lavender essential oil on your pillowcase or in a diffuser can create a serene sleep environment. If lavender isn't your thing, other relaxing oils like chamomile, ylang-ylang, or cedarwood can also be effective. These natural scents can help trigger your brain's relaxation response, fostering a more restful night (Conrad & Adams, 2012).

We can't overlook the power of a warm bath. Soaking in a tub filled with warm water can help ease muscle tension, and adding Epsom salts can provide additional stress relief. Magnesium in the Epsom salts can be absorbed through the skin, promoting muscle relaxation and reducing stress. Try incorporating calming elements like candles, dim lighting, and perhaps a few drops of lavender oil to enhance the experience. The warmth of the water can even help regulate your body's temperature, encouraging you to fall asleep faster (Michaels, 2021).

Guided imagery is another technique worth exploring. This method involves using mental images to influence how you feel emotionally and physically. Essentially, you close your eyes and imagine yourself in a peaceful, serene setting—perhaps a quiet beach or a calm forest. Focus on the sensory experiences you'd encounter there: the sound of the waves, the smell of the pine trees, the feeling of cool sand underfoot. Guided imagery can shift your focus away from stress and anxiety, lulling you into a more relaxed state conducive to sleep.

Acupressure, though less commonly discussed, can also be a beneficial relaxation technique. Similar to acupuncture but without the needles, acupressure involves applying pressure to specific points on the body to relieve tension and promote relaxation. Common points that can help alleviate stress include the area between your eyebrows, the point between your thumb and forefinger, and the inside of your wrist. Applying gentle, consistent pressure to these points for a few minutes can activate your body's natural relaxation response, making it easier to slip into sleep (Zick et al., 2008).

Yoga, often celebrated for its physical benefits, also excels in stress reduction and promoting better sleep. Specific poses like Child's Pose, Legs-Up-The-Wall, and Corpse Pose are designed to relax the body and calm the mind. Incorporate gentle, mindful movements with a focus on deep, rhythmic breathing. Engaging in a short yoga session before bedtime can help release physical and emotional tension, setting the stage for improved sleep quality (Chang et al., 2016).

Journaling is a practice I highly recommend to many of my clients struggling with sleep due to stress. Writing down your thoughts and feelings before bed can act as a release, helping to get worries and anxieties out of your head and onto paper. It doesn't have to be anything formal—just a brain dump of what's been on your mind. This simple act can help calm a racing mind, making it easier to transition to sleep. Some people find it helpful to jot down a few things they're grateful for as well, which can shift your focus to more positive thoughts.

Lastly, don't underestimate the value of a bedtime routine. Engaging in the same calming activities each night can create a sense of comfort and predictability, which can be very soothing. Whether it's reading a book, sipping on a cup of herbal tea, or spending a few minutes in meditation, a consistent routine can signal to your brain that it's time to wind down and prepare for sleep. Consistency is key here—try to follow your bedtime routine at the same time each night to help regulate your internal clock.

If you're struggling with sleep, it's essential to experiment with different relaxation techniques to find what works best for you. Everyone's different, and what works wonders for one person might not be as effective for another. It's about building a toolkit of strategies that you can draw on whenever you need to de-stress and prepare for a good night's rest. Keep an open mind and be willing to try new approaches until you find the perfect combination that lets you sleep soundly.

Incorporating these relaxation techniques into your daily routine isn't just about improving your sleep—it's about enhancing your overall well-being. Reduced stress levels can lead to improved mental health, better physical health, and an overall higher quality of life. So, give these techniques a try, see what resonates with you, and take one step closer to achieving the restful, restorative sleep you deserve.

Mindfulness and Meditation

Let's dive into the realm of mindfulness and meditation, two simple yet powerful allies in your quest for better sleep. At first glance, they may seem like trendy buzzwords, but the science behind their effectiveness is both compelling and robust. For the perpetually stressed-out professional or the overworked student, mastering mindfulness and meditation can make all the difference between tossing and turning or enjoying peaceful, restorative sleep.

Mindfulness refers to the practice of being present in the moment, aware of your thoughts, feelings, and surroundings without judgment. It's about grounding yourself in the here and now, rather than being caught up in past regrets or future anxieties. When it comes to sleep, mindfulness can be particularly effective in breaking the cycle of stress and insomnia. Research has shown that mindfulness meditation can significantly reduce symptoms of insomnia and improve overall sleep quality (Black et al., 2015).

But how exactly does this work? When practiced consistently, mindfulness rewires the brain in a way that enhances your ability to manage stress. The prefrontal cortex, the area of the brain responsible for executive functions like decision-making and emotional regulation, becomes more active. Meanwhile, the amygdala, which is responsible for triggering the stress response, shows reduced activity (Hölzel et al.,

2011). This shift helps create a state of calm that is conducive to falling asleep and staying asleep.

If you've never tried meditation before, you might feel a bit skeptical about its benefits. After all, sitting still and doing nothing doesn't exactly sound like a radical solution to your sleep problems. But the essence of meditation is far from doing nothing. It's an active practice that trains your mind to focus, relax, and let go of troubling thoughts.

Consider starting with simple mindfulness meditation. Find a quiet spot, sit comfortably, and close your eyes. Start by focusing on your breath—notice the inhale, the brief pause, and the exhale. When your mind inevitably starts to wander, gently bring your focus back to your breath. It's all about returning to the present moment, over and over again. Even just five to ten minutes a day can make a noticeable difference.

For those nights when anxiety robs you of sleep, another helpful technique is the body scan meditation. This involves mentally scanning your body from head to toe, paying attention to any sensations of tension or discomfort. By acknowledging and releasing this tension, you create an optimal environment for sleep. A study conducted by the American Academy of Sleep Medicine found that participants who practiced body scan meditation experienced significant improvements in sleep quality (Ong et al., 2014).

Guided meditations can also be a fantastic way to ease into the practice. Numerous apps (think Headspace, Calm, and Insight Timer) offer guided sessions specifically designed to help you unwind and prepare for sleep. These usually combine breathing exercises with soothing narratives, making it easier for you to let go of the day's stress and drift into slumber.

Beyond traditional sitting meditation, incorporating mindfulness into your daily activities can also be beneficial. Whether you're eating, walking, or even brushing your teeth, try to be fully present. Notice the texture, smell, and taste of your food. Pay attention to the sensation of your feet hitting the ground. By cultivating mindfulness throughout the day, you're setting the groundwork for a more relaxed mind come bedtime.

Now, you might be wondering about the time commitment involved. The beauty of mindfulness and meditation is that they are incredibly flexible. While it's great if you can manage a 20-minute session, shorter periods are also effective. The key is consistency. Just like physical exercise, the benefits of mindfulness and meditation compound over time. A few minutes every day is better than longer sessions once in a while.

Moreover, mindfulness isn't just about improving sleep—it's a holistic lifestyle change. It fosters a greater sense of well-being and equips you with tools for emotional resilience. This can have a ripple effect, improving other aspects of your life that, in turn, contribute to better sleep. For instance, managing work stress more effectively can reduce those 3 AM jolt-awake moments when all your to-dos flood your mind.

It's also worth noting that mindfulness and meditation can work in conjunction with other relaxation techniques. Progressive muscle relaxation, deep breathing exercises, and even light yoga can complement your mindfulness practice, creating a well-rounded strategy for stress reduction and improved sleep.

One thing to keep top of mind: patience. Don't expect overnight results. Like any skill, meditation takes time to cultivate. But rest assured, the benefits you'll reap are well worth the effort. Not only will you likely experience better sleep, but you'll also notice improvements in focus, creativity, and overall emotional well-being.

As you embark on this journey, remember that there's no "right" or "wrong" way to practice mindfulness and meditation. It's a highly personal experience. What works for one person might not resonate with another. Feel free to adapt and experiment until you find what best suits your lifestyle and needs.

In summary, the integration of mindfulness and meditation into your daily routine can be transformative. From rewiring your brain to handle stress better to fostering an environment conducive to restful sleep, these practices hold significant promise. And while the path to mastering them might be gradual, the positive impact on your health and well-being is undeniable. Make them a part of your nightly wind-down, and you might just find that sleep comes a little easier, and stress's grip loosens a bit more each night.

Chapter 9:
Exercise and Sleep

Exercise holds the key to unlocking a more restful night's sleep, providing both an immediate sense of relaxation and long-term benefits for sleep quality and overall health. Engaging in regular physical activity helps to regulate your body's internal clock, also known as the circadian rhythm, making it easier to fall asleep and wake up at consistent times (Myllymäki et al., 2012). Not all exercise is created equal in its sleep-enhancing properties; moderate aerobic activities like walking or swimming may be the most beneficial (Kredlow et al., 2015). Moreover, the timing of exercise plays a crucial role—exercising too close to bedtime can sometimes have a stimulating effect, making it harder to drift off to sleep (Buman & King, 2010). Nevertheless, incorporating exercise into your daily routine can significantly reduce symptoms of insomnia and sleep apnea by improving sleep efficiency and reducing the time it takes to fall asleep. While more research is needed to understand the exact mechanisms, the consensus is clear: making exercise a habitual part of your day can pave the way to more restorative sleep.

Best Times to Exercise

Let's face it—fitting exercise into an already jam-packed schedule is no small feat. We all know that working out is a cornerstone of a healthy lifestyle, complementing our dietary habits and mental well-being. But did you know the timing of your physical activity could make or break your sleep quality? It's all about finding that sweet spot in your day that maximizes your exercise benefits while ensuring you get the restful sleep you deserve.

If you're someone who likes to rise with the sun, morning workouts might just be your saving grace. Exercising in the morning might set a positive tone for the rest of your day. A study published in *Sleep Medicine* found that morning exercise can help regulate your circadian rhythm (Youngstedt et al., 2002). This makes it easier to fall asleep at night because it aligns your physical activity with your body's natural sleep-wake cycle. Plus, the boost in endorphins and adrenaline can make you more productive throughout the day.

Afternoon workouts, typically between 1 PM and 4 PM, can also be incredibly beneficial for sleep. During these hours, your body temperature is naturally higher, meaning your muscles are more flexible, and you're more energetic. According to a study from *Chronobiology International*, exercising in the late afternoon can improve sleep efficiency more effectively than morning or evening workouts (Baehr et al., 2003). This time slot is especially useful for those who want a strong performance in their workouts without potentially interrupting their nightly rest.

When it comes to evening exercise, things get a bit more nuanced. There's a common belief that working out too late can keep you wired and sleepless, but this isn't universally true. Research has shown that moderate to vigorous evening exercise doesn't necessarily impede sleep. A study in *Sports Medicine* suggests that it depends on the individual and the intensity of the workout (Myllymaki et al., 2011). While some people can do high-intensity interval training (HIIT) at 8 PM without any repercussions, others might feel restless and have difficulty winding down.

Timing isn't the only factor to consider; the type of exercise also plays a crucial role. For example, high-intensity workouts should ideally be reserved for earlier in the day. High-adrenaline activities like sprinting or heavy weightlifting can elevate your heart rate and body temperature, potentially making it harder to transition into a calm, restful state at bedtime. On the other hand, low-intensity exercises like yoga or stretching routines can be more suitable for the evening. These activities not only help in muscle recovery but also promote relaxation, making it easier for you to fall asleep.

Let's not ignore the role of hormones in this equation. Exercising, particularly during the daytime, boosts the secretion of serotonin and reduces cortisol levels. By balancing these hormones, you're likely to experience less stress and anxiety, making it easier to drift off to sleep. Jessica Matthews from the *American Council on Exercise* notes that regular exercise has a profound effect on sleep patterns, primarily by increasing the time spent in deep sleep phases where restorative processes occur (Matthews, 2015).

However, let's not kid ourselves—various factors can influence the best time for you to exercise, from your daily schedule to personal preferences. What works for one person may not work for another. Your job routine, family responsibilities, and social commitments all come into play here. That's why it's crucial to experiment and find what fits seamlessly into your life.

Even adjusting your meal timings can complement your workout schedule. Eating a nutritious breakfast post-morning exercise can fuel your day. In contrast, a balanced dinner post-evening workout can expedite muscle recovery. Furthermore, make sure to stay hydrated throughout the day to maintain optimal performance and recovery.

Speaking of hydration, dehydration can seriously impair both your exercise performance and sleep quality. According to a study published in the *Journal of Clinical Sleep Medicine*, even mild dehydration can negatively impact your sleep duration and efficiency (Snyder et al.,

2012). Therefore, make it a habit to drink plenty of water, regardless of when you decide to hit the gym.

An often overlooked but equally vital aspect is consistency. Sporadically shifting your workout times can disrupt your body's internal clock, leading to irregular sleep patterns. It's far more beneficial to stick to a regular exercise schedule. Consistency helps your body predict and adjust, making it easier to achieve that restful slumber every night.

While we're on the subject of consistency, let's talk about the importance of listening to your body. Being attuned to your body's signals can guide you in figuring out the optimal time for your workouts. Are you more alert and energetic in the morning? Then morning exercises might be your best bet. Alternatively, if you find your energy peaking in the late afternoon, capitalize on that time slot for your physical activity.

Lastly, don't underestimate the power of small but consistent changes. Even if you can't find a full hour to exercise, short 15-20 minute workout bursts throughout the day can still improve your overall health and sleep quality. According to a study in *Frontiers in Physiology*, these micro-workouts can be just as effective when looked at cumulatively over the week (Gibala et al., 2016). This approach can be particularly helpful for those juggling multiple responsibilities yet striving for a healthier lifestyle.

In conclusion, the best time to exercise largely depends on your personal circumstances, including your work schedule, family obligations, and natural energy cycles. Morning workouts can help you seize the day, afternoon sessions optimize performance and sleep efficiency, and evening exercises can be beneficial if they're of lower intensity. Remember, the key is consistency and listening to your body. With a balanced approach, you can find the perfect workout rhythm that not only fits your lifestyle but significantly improves your sleep quality.

Types of Exercise for Better Sleep

When it comes to getting better sleep, not all exercises are created equal. The type of physical activity you choose can have a significant impact on how well you rest at night. Let's dive into some of the best types of exercise that can help you achieve better sleep, how they work, and why they're effective.

First up, we have aerobic or "cardio" exercise. This includes activities such as running, cycling, swimming, and even brisk walking. Aerobic exercise has been shown to improve sleep quality significantly. Engaging in regular cardio can help reduce the time it takes to fall asleep and increase the total sleep duration (Reid et al., 2010). One reason for this is that cardio exercises elevate your heart rate for an extended period, which helps to reduce stress and anxiety, making it easier for your mind to wind down at night.

Strength training, also known as resistance training, can also be a valuable asset in your sleep-improvement toolkit. This type of exercise encompasses weightlifting, bodyweight exercises like push-ups and squats, and using resistance bands. A study by Misra and colleagues (2015) found that people who included strength training in their routines fell asleep faster and enjoyed deeper sleep compared to those who did not engage in such activities. Strength training contributes to better sleep by improving your overall physical health, which includes balanced hormone levels that regulate sleep patterns.

Flexibility and balance exercises are often overlooked but play a crucial role in improving sleep. Yoga and stretching exercises fall into this category. Yoga, in particular, has been shown to be extremely beneficial for improving sleep quality. A systematic review of multiple studies concluded that yoga can decrease the severity of insomnia and improve overall sleep efficiency (Cramer et al., 2017). The meditative aspects of yoga help reduce stress, while the physical postures relieve tension accumulated in the body, thereby paving the way for a restful night.

High-intensity interval training (HIIT) may be another option worth considering. Although HIIT workouts are shorter in duration, they can be very effective in improving sleep. This type of exercise involves short bursts of intense activity followed by a period of rest or low-intensity exercise. Research has shown that HIIT can improve the quality of slow-wave sleep, the deepest stage of sleep, which is critical for physical recovery and overall well-being (Wood & Reilly, 2018). However, timing matters for HIIT; it's generally best to perform these exercises earlier in the day to avoid overstimulation close to bedtime.

It's essential to mention that different people may respond differently to various types of exercise. For some, a long session of moderate-intensity exercise in the evening can be calming, while for others, it can be stimulating and make it harder to fall asleep. Listening to your body and observing how it reacts to different types of exercise at various times of day can provide valuable insights into what works best for you.

While these different types of exercises all have their merits, consistency is key. Regular physical activity is the overarching theme that ties these various forms of exercise together. Whether you prefer aerobics, strength training, flexibility exercises, or HIIT, making exercise a regular part of your routine is what will yield the most significant improvements in sleep quality.

Incorporating exercise into your daily routine doesn't have to be a monumental task. You might start with something as simple as a 20-minute walk in the evening or a quick yoga session before bed. What's essential is finding an activity that you enjoy so that it becomes a sustainable habit, rather than a chore.

Moreover, the timing of your exercise can also play a role. There is much debate about the optimal time to exercise for better sleep. Generally speaking, exercising in the afternoon or early evening can be beneficial. A study showed that engaging in physical activity at these times could help people fall asleep faster and sleep more soundly (Passos et al., 2010). The research suggests that timing your workouts too close to bedtime might have the opposite effect, making it harder to wind down.

Lastly, while vigorous exercise has its benefits, don't underestimate the power of light or moderate activities. Even something as simple as gardening or a leisurely bike ride can improve your sleep. These activities reduce stress hormones and increase the production of sleep-promoting hormones like melatonin.

In conclusion, achieving better sleep through exercise is not about finding a one-size-fits-all solution but rather discovering what works best for you. A mix of aerobic, strength, flexibility, and even HIIT exercises can be your go-to arsenal for fighting sleep problems. Regularity, enjoyment, and appropriate timing are your guiding principles. As you experiment with different types of exercise, you will inevitably find the right balance that helps you achieve the restful sleep you deserve.

Chapter 10:
Developing a Sleep Routine

Let's dive right into the cornerstone of great sleep: developing a consistent sleep routine. Consistency is a game-changer when it comes to sleep, as it helps regulate your body's internal clock, otherwise known as the circadian rhythm (Czeisler et al., 1999). A well-structured sleep routine sets the stage for your body to know exactly when it's time to wind down and wake up. Start by setting a regular sleep and wake time, even on weekends. This might feel challenging initially, but your body will thank you in the long run. Incorporate pre-sleep rituals like dimming the lights, turning off electronic devices, and engaging in calming activities such as reading or taking a warm bath (Chang et al., 2015). These rituals signal to your brain that it's time to relax and prepare for sleep. Over time, these small changes can significantly improve your sleep quality and overall well-being (Walker, 2017). No magic formula here, just dedication and understanding that better sleep is a marathon, not a sprint.

The Power of Consistency

Imagine waking up every morning feeling refreshed and ready to conquer your day. It sounds like a dream, but it's more within your grasp than you might think. The magic ingredient? Consistency. When it comes to developing a sleep routine, the power of consistency can't be overstated. Our bodies thrive on routine, and establishing a consistent sleep schedule is key to unlocking better sleep quality.

You see, our bodies have something called a circadian rhythm—a natural, internal process that regulates the sleep-wake cycle and repeats roughly every 24 hours (Czeisler, 1999). This biological clock is heavily influenced by external cues, the most significant being light. By going to bed and waking up at the same time every day, you're essentially programming your circadian rhythm, making it easier for your body to know when to wind down for sleep and when to wake up.

Let's not sugarcoat it—adjusting to a consistent sleep routine isn't always straightforward. There will be late-night parties, work emergencies, and Netflix binges that will tempt you to stay up past your bedtime. This is where the challenge lies. However, the benefits of adhering to a regular sleep schedule far outweigh the occasional sacrifice. For one, a consistent sleep pattern improves sleep quality. When your body knows what to expect, it can optimize the time you spend in deep sleep and REM stages, which are crucial for cognitive functions such as memory consolidation and emotional regulation (Walker, 2017).

Moreover, consistency isn't just about the timing of your sleep; it also involves creating a stable pre-sleep routine. Engaging in relaxing activities before bed—like reading, meditating, or gentle stretching—can signal to your body that it's time to sleep. Over time, these activities become cues that help you transition smoothly from wakefulness to sleep. When you have a set bedtime routine, you're less likely to find yourself tossing and turning, struggling to fall asleep.

One important aspect of maintaining a consistent sleep schedule is addressing sleep hygiene. Sleep hygiene refers to the practices and habits that promote good quality sleep. This includes creating a conducive sleep environment, limiting caffeine and alcohol intake before bed, and keeping a cool and dark bedroom. But here's the catch: these practices are most effective when they're applied consistently.

Sporadic efforts will get you nowhere. It's the daily commitment to these habits that will yield the best results.

For those who find themselves traveling frequently or working irregular shifts, maintaining a consistent sleep schedule can be particularly challenging. However, it's not impossible. You might need to be a bit more flexible in these situations, but even small efforts to keep your sleep timing regular can make a big difference. Some strategies include using blackout curtains to manage light exposure, taking short naps to adjust your sleep debt, and employing relaxation techniques to help you fall asleep more quickly.

Scientific evidence strongly supports the benefits of a consistent sleep schedule. Studies have shown correlations between irregular sleep patterns and a host of health issues, ranging from metabolic disorders to mental health problems (Roenneberg et al., 2012). Irregular sleep can disrupt the body's metabolism, making you more susceptible to gaining weight and developing conditions like diabetes. It can also impact your mood and cognitive performance, leading to symptoms of anxiety and depression. By sticking to a regular sleep schedule, you're actively supporting your overall health and well-being.

Achieving consistency in your sleep routine also involves understanding your own body's needs. Everyone's sleep requirements are different. Some of us thrive on seven hours of sleep, while others might need a full nine hours to feel their best. The key is to find out what works best for you and stick to it. Keeping a sleep diary can be incredibly helpful in identifying your sleep patterns and pinpointing what disruptions need to be addressed. Once you've nailed down what works, making consistency a priority becomes much easier.

It's also worth mentioning the social aspect of sleep consistency. When you commit to a regular sleep schedule, you might have to navigate social pressures. Friends and family might not understand why you're turning down late-night plans or why you're adamant about waking up early on weekends. However, staying true to your sleep routine is an investment in your health. Over time, those around you might even become inspired by your commitment and join you in adopting healthier sleep habits.

Lastly, one of the most significant perks of maintaining a consistent sleep routine is the predictability it brings to your day-to-day life. When your sleep schedule is stable, you can plan your activities more effectively and be more productive. Your energy levels will be more consistent, and you'll find it easier to concentrate and remain focused throughout the day. It's a win-win situation.

If you're ready to harness the power of consistency in your sleep routine, start with small, manageable changes. Gradually adjust your bedtime by 15-minute increments until you reach your desired sleep schedule. Maintain this timing every day—even on weekends. Consistency might feel monotonous, but remember, it's the key that unlocks the door to better sleep and, ultimately, a higher quality of life.

Pre-Sleep Rituals

Think of pre-sleep rituals as your personal wind-down routine, designed to signal to your brain that it's time to slow down and prepare for sleep. Our bodies thrive on consistency because of the internal body clock, or circadian rhythm, which regulates the sleep-wake cycle. Before you toss and turn wondering why you can't fall asleep, consider how a lack of consistent pre-sleep rituals might be the culprit.

First things first, let's talk about timing. Establishing a regular bedtime isn't just for kids; it's crucial for adults, too. Aim to go to bed and wake up at the same time every day—even on weekends. Disruptions to this schedule can affect your ability to fall asleep and stay asleep (Hirshkowitz et al., 2015). This consistency is the cornerstone of any effective pre-sleep ritual, so make it a non-negotiable part of your routine.

Now, once you've established a consistent bedtime, the wind-down process can begin. Start by creating a calming environment. Dim the lights in your living areas about an hour before bed. Our bodies are sensitive to light, which can impact the production of melatonin, the hormone responsible for regulating sleep (Gooley et al., 2011). Lowering the lights signals to your body that it's time for relaxation and rest.

Consider incorporating a specific activity that helps you unwind. Reading a book can be a great way to signal your brain that it's time to relax—but steer clear of action-packed novels or intense non-fiction. Go for something calming, like poetry or light fiction. Alternatively, mindfulness practices such as meditation or deep breathing exercises can do wonders. Studies show that these practices can significantly reduce stress levels, making it easier to fall asleep (Winbush, Gross, & Kreitzer, 2007).

A warm bath around 90 minutes before bedtime is another fantastic pre-sleep ritual. The science here is fascinating: when you take a warm bath, your body's core temperature increases. After exiting the bath, your body temperature begins to drop, mimicking the natural decline in core temperature that happens before sleep (Murphy et al., 1997). This can help you drift off more easily.

Next, let's not underestimate the power of scent. Aromatherapy, particularly using lavender essential oil, has been proven to improve sleep quality (Lewith, Godfrey, & Prescott, 2005). A simple ritual could be to diffuse lavender oil in your bedroom or dab a bit on your pillow. This small addition to your nightly routine can substantially impact your ability to relax and fall asleep.

Of course, what you drink matters. Caffeine is the enemy of good sleep, so avoid it at least four to six hours before bedtime (Drake et al., 2013). Instead, opt for a calming herbal tea, like chamomile, known for its mild sedative effects. Avoid alcohol as well; while it might make you sleepy at first, it disrupts your sleep cycle, leading to poorer sleep quality overall (Roehrs & Roth, 2001).

Another powerful ritual is the practice of journaling. Spending just 5-10 minutes writing down your thoughts can help you offload any lingering worries or to-do lists cluttering your mind. Research indicates that expressive writing before bedtime can significantly reduce pre-sleep cognitive arousal, facilitating an easier transition to sleep (Harvey & Farrell, 2003).

Acoustic stimulation can also play a role. Listening to calming music or white noise before bed can help signal to your body that it's time to wind down. A study found that participants who listened to soothing music before bed experienced better sleep quality than those who didn't (Harmat et al., 2008). Whether it's nature sounds, classical music, or a white noise machine, find what works best for you.

Lastly, ensure you keep your bedtime digital-free. Ignoring this can make all other pre-sleep rituals ineffective. Blue light emitted from phones, tablets, and computers can trick our brains into thinking it's daytime, thus delaying melatonin production (Chang et al., 2015). Make it a rule to ditch the digital devices at least an hour before bed. Instead, indulge in one of the other suggested rituals.

In summary, developing pre-sleep rituals involves a combination of consistency, environmental changes, and specific relaxing activities. Incorporate a few of these strategies into your evening routine to find what works best for you. The key is to make these rituals consistent and non-negotiable; the more regular you are, the better your sleep quality will be. Remember, preparing for sleep should be a cherished part of your day that you look forward to, not a chore. So take these tips to heart, and you might find yourself sleeping better than you ever thought possible.

Chapter 11:
Understanding Sleep Aids

When insomnia hits, navigating the diverse landscape of sleep aids can seem daunting. Over-the-counter options like melatonin and antihistamines are popular starting points, but it's crucial to understand their mechanisms and potential side effects (Kolla et al., 2018). While melatonin, often dubbed the "sleep hormone," can help regulate your circadian rhythm, it's not a long-term fix and is best used for occasional sleeplessness or jet lag (Costello et al., 2014). On the natural side, herbal supplements such as valerian root and chamomile have shown promise in promoting relaxation and improved sleep (Fernández-San-Martín et al., 2010). However, it's essential to consult a healthcare provider before diving into any sleep aid regimen to ensure it aligns with your unique health landscape. Ultimately, understanding the pros and cons of these options can empower you to make informed choices tailored to your needs, paving the way for restful nights and rejuvenated mornings.

Over-the-Counter Options

When you're running on fumes and looking for a quick fix to get some much-needed shut-eye, a stroll down the pharmacy aisle might seem like the simplest solution. Over-the-counter sleep aids offer a tempting reprieve from those sleepless nights, promising restful sleep in the form of pills, liquids, or gummies. While these options may provide temporary relief, it's crucial to understand their effects, efficacy, and potential risks.

Firstly, it's essential to recognize that most over-the-counter sleep aids fall into two main categories: antihistamines and melatonin supplements. Antihistamines, such as diphenhydramine (found in Benadryl and many nighttime cold medications) and doxylamine (found in Unisom), are primarily developed to treat allergies. However, one of their side effects is drowsiness, making them popular as short-term sleep solutions (Kuriyama et al., 2014).

Antihistamines work by blocking histamine receptors in the brain. Histamines play a key role in wakefulness and, when blocked, can make you feel sleepy. However, while effective at inducing sleep, these medications often come with a host of side effects, including dry mouth, dizziness, and next-day drowsiness. More alarmingly, frequent use can lead to tolerance, meaning you may need higher doses to achieve the same effect over time—a scenario that risks dependency without addressing the underlying problem (Richardson et al., 2002).

Melatonin supplements are another common over-the-counter option. Melatonin is a hormone that your body naturally produces in response to darkness, helping regulate your sleep-wake cycle. It's often marketed as a natural solution for sleep issues, and research indicates it can be effective, especially for certain conditions like jet lag and shift work disorder (Wright et al., 2012). The appeal of melatonin lies in its role in synchronizing the circadian rhythm, making it particularly useful for situations where this rhythm is disrupted.

However, it's important to be cautious with dosages and timing. Unlike prescription medications, melatonin supplements are not as strictly regulated, meaning the concentration listed on the bottle might not always be what you're getting. Too much melatonin can actually disrupt your sleep cycle further, leading to issues like vivid dreams or grogginess the next day. Generally, smaller doses (0.5 mg to 3 mg) are recommended and should be taken a couple of hours before bedtime to mimic the body's natural melatonin production (Elder et al., 2012).

What about herbal remedies? Over-the-counter shelves are also filled with products like valerian root, chamomile, and lavender, all hailed for their supposed sleep-inducing properties. Valerian root, for example, has been used for centuries as a remedy for insomnia and anxiety. Some studies suggest it may help improve sleep quality and reduce the time it takes to fall asleep, though results are mixed and more research is needed (Fernandez-San-Martin et al., 2010).

Chamomile tea is another popular choice; its calming effects are often attributed to an antioxidant called apigenin, which binds to receptors in the brain that promote relaxation. Lavender, generally used in aromatherapy, is known for its soothing properties, and some evidence suggests it can improve feelings of well-being and sleep quality when used as an essential oil (Herz, 2009). However, while these herbal remedies come with fewer side effects, they may not be as potent or fast-acting as pharmaceutical options.

One critical aspect to remember is that over-the-counter sleep aids are generally meant for short-term use. They aren't designed to address chronic sleep disorders or severe insomnia. If you find yourself relying on these aids more frequently, it may be time to consult a healthcare professional. Chronic sleep problems often indicate underlying health issues that need to be addressed with a more comprehensive approach.

Moreover, relying heavily on these aids can sometimes mask the behaviors that are contributing to poor sleep in the first place. For instance, poor sleep hygiene, such as inconsistent sleep schedules, excessive caffeine or alcohol intake, and overuse of electronic devices, can significantly affect your ability to fall and stay asleep. Tackling these behaviors head-on is often a more effective and sustainable solution.

It's also worth noting that while over-the-counter sleep aids are readily accessible, they're not free of risks. Apart from the potential side effects and dependency issues discussed earlier, there's the danger of drug interactions if you're taking other medications. Always read labels carefully and consider speaking with a pharmacist or doctor to ensure that an over-the-counter sleep aid won't conflict with any other treatments you're undergoing.

Lastly, it can be empowering to know that achieving better sleep doesn't always have to come from a bottle. By implementing some of the strategies discussed in other sections of this book—such as optimizing your sleep environment, managing stress, and establishing a consistent sleep routine—you might find you don't need to rely on over-the-counter solutions as much as you thought.

In the end, if you decide to use over-the-counter sleep aids, do so with a well-informed approach, understanding their benefits and limitations. Treat them as a short-term bridge to better sleep habits, not as a long-term crutch. After all, the ultimate goal here is to empower you with the knowledge and tools to achieve consistently restful and rejuvenating sleep, night after night.

Natural Alternatives

When it comes to sleep aids, many of us instinctively reach for over-the-counter solutions, but natural alternatives offer a plethora of benefits without the risk of dependency or unwanted side effects. Integrating these into your routine may support better sleep naturally while also optimizing overall health and well-being.

First and foremost, valerian root is one of the most widely recognized natural sleep aids. Derived from the valerian plant, it's particularly celebrated for its calming effect and ability to reduce the time it takes to fall asleep. Unlike some prescription medications, valerian root doesn't leave you feeling groggy the next day (Bent et al.,

2006). It's available in various forms, including capsules, teas, and tinctures, making it easy to incorporate into your nightly routine.

Another effective option is melatonin, a hormone that your body naturally produces to regulate sleep-wake cycles. Melatonin supplements can be particularly helpful for individuals dealing with jet lag or shift work. While it's a natural hormone, it's essential to use it judiciously under the guidance of a healthcare provider to avoid disrupting your body's natural production (Zhdanova et al., 2001). Recommended doses typically range from 0.5 to 5 milligrams, taken 30 to 60 minutes before bed.

Chamomile tea is another age-old remedy praised for its sleep-inducing properties. Beyond sleep, chamomile has anti-inflammatory, antimicrobial, and antioxidant properties, making it a great choice for overall well-being (Srivastava et al., 2010). A calming cup of chamomile before bed can help you unwind and prepare your body for restful sleep.

Lavender, both in essential oil form and as a tea, can significantly impact sleep quality. Lavender essential oil can be diffused in your bedroom, added to a relaxing bath, or applied topically to further enhance its calming effects. Studies show that lavender can enhance deep sleep, helping you wake up feeling refreshed and more alert (Koulivand et al., 2013).

Another natural solution worth exploring is magnesium. This essential mineral plays a crucial role in numerous bodily functions, including muscle relaxation. A deficiency can lead to symptoms like insomnia and restless sleep. Magnesium supplements or magnesium-rich foods like leafy greens and nuts can help improve sleep quality significantly (Abbasi et al., 2012).

For some, the simple act of sipping on a glass of warm milk before bed can evoke feelings of comfort and relaxation. This is not just an old wives' tale; milk contains tryptophan, an amino acid that the body converts into serotonin and melatonin, both of which are essential for sleep regulation.

Other lesser-known but effective natural sleep aids include passionflower and lemon balm. Passionflower, particularly as a tea, can help with sleep disturbances related to stress and anxiety (Akhondzadeh et al., 2001). Lemon balm, when taken as a supplement or tea, has been shown to significantly improve sleep parameters, including time taken to fall asleep and sleep quality (Kennedy et al., 2006).

While trying these natural alternatives, it's important to remind oneself that consistency is key. Integrating these solutions into a nightly ritual can often yield better results than sporadically using them. It's about creating a holistic approach toward winding down and preparing the mind and body for rest.

It's also worth noting that natural doesn't always mean risk-free. Always consult with a healthcare provider before starting any new supplement, especially if you're pregnant, nursing, or taking other medications. Some herbs can interact with other medications and may not be suitable for everyone.

Incorporating these natural remedies can provide a gentler, more holistic approach to improving sleep. They often come with the added benefit of supporting overall wellness, making it easier to achieve a restful night's sleep without the unwanted side effects sometimes associated with over-the-counter medications.

Chapter 12:
The Special Cases: Shift Workers and Frequent Travelers

Life doesn't adhere to a 9-to-5 schedule for everyone, and shift workers and frequent travelers often find themselves wrestling with disruptive sleep patterns. Shift workers, who toil through graveyard shifts or rotating schedules, frequently face a circadian rhythm misalignment, which can lead to chronic sleep deprivation and a host of health issues (Saksvik et al., 2011). On the other hand, frequent travelers battle jet lag, a temporary circadian rhythm disorder characterized by misalignment between the internal body clock and the local time (Arendt, 2009). This chapter dives into effective strategies tailored for these special cases to restore balance and ensure quality sleep. From optimizing light exposure and employing strategic naps to understanding the benefits of melatonin for resetting internal clocks, we've got you covered with science-backed recommendations to navigate these unique challenges. Remember, small adjustments can make a massive difference in achieving restorative sleep, even when life throws you off the usual sleep track.

Tips for Shift Workers

If you're working shifts, you probably know firsthand how challenging it can be to get quality sleep. From irregular hours to trying to sleep during daylight, shift work introduces a unique set of problems that can mess up your natural sleep rhythm. But don't worry, there are effective ways to mitigate these challenges and get better rest, even if your schedule feels like it was designed by an evil wizard.

First things first: understanding your body's circadian rhythm is vital. Your circadian rhythm is basically your internal clock, which runs on a roughly 24-hour cycle and dictates when you feel awake and when you feel sleepy. Regular shifts can throw this completely out of whack. To align your internal clock as much as possible, establish a consistent sleep schedule—even on your days off. This helps your body know what to expect, which can promote more restful sleep. Furthermore, consider using blackout curtains and eye masks to simulate nighttime, making it easier to fall asleep during daylight hours.

When you're working night shifts, taking a strategic nap can be a game-changer. A short nap of about 20-30 minutes can help you stay alert and maintain performance during your shift. In fact, naps enhance alertness and performance better than caffeine (Brooks & Lack, 2006). Just make sure not to nap too close to your main sleep time, as this can make it harder to fall asleep later.

Notably, diet plays a critical role in your ability to maintain alertness and restfulness. Avoid heavy meals before bed since they can cause discomfort and disrupt sleep. Instead, opt for light snacks like a banana or a small bowl of oatmeal, which are easier to digest and can even promote sleep due to their natural melatonin content (e.g., bananas). Also, try to time your caffeine intake so that it doesn't interfere with your sleep. Remember, caffeine can stay in your system for up to 6 hours (Bonnet & Arand, 1992), so plan your last cup accordingly.

You might be wondering about the role of physical activity for shift workers. Incorporating regular exercise into your daily routine can improve overall sleep quality. However, timing is crucial. Exercising too close to bedtime can make it harder to wind down, while moderate exercise earlier in the day can be beneficial (Driver & Taylor, 2000).

Your work environment also plays a role. If your work setting allows, try to expose yourself to bright light during your shift. Bright light can help trick your body into staying awake and alert. Conversely, reduce light exposure as you near the end of your shift to signal your brain that it's time to wind down. Portable light boxes can be used to enhance light exposure during night shifts, while blue light-blocking glasses can be handy when you're heading home and need to prepare for sleep.

Creating a pre-sleep routine is another essential strategy. Develop calming activities before bed, like reading a book, listening to soft music, or practicing relaxation techniques such as deep breathing exercises. These actions cue your body that it's time to wind down, making it easier to transition to sleep.

For some, making use of natural sleep aids like melatonin supplements can be beneficial. Melatonin, a hormone that your body naturally produces to regulate sleep-wake cycles, has been shown to improve sleep quality in shift workers (Arendt et al., 1997). Before introducing any supplements into your regimen, consult your healthcare provider to ensure they're appropriate for you.

Shift workers often juggle the urge to socialize on regular schedules while also handling their irregular work hours. Striking a balance is key. While it's important not to isolate yourself, prioritize your rest as well. Communicate with friends and family about your schedule; they'll likely be more understanding when they know you're aiming to prioritize your health.

Furthermore, creating an optimal sleep environment is critical for shift workers. This means investing in a comfortable mattress and pillows, ensuring the room is cool (around 65°F), and minimizing noise disruptions using earplugs or white noise machines. Making your sleep environment as inviting and restful as possible can significantly increase the quality of your sleep, even if it's during unconventional hours.

Let's touch on one crucial aspect—mental health. It can be easy to overlook, but continuously missing out on good sleep can have a cascading effect on your mental health. Being proactive about managing stress through mindfulness techniques like meditation can have a significant impact. Regular mindfulness practice has been associated with better sleep quality and duration (Black et al., 2015).

Finally, staying hydrated is often overlooked but equally important. Dehydration can lead to feelings of fatigue, so make sure you're drinking enough water throughout your shift and before bed. Just be cautious not to drink too much water right before you hit the sack to avoid multiple bathroom trips interrupting your precious sleep.

Shift work can feel like navigating a minefield of sleep challenges, but equipped with the right strategies, you can significantly improve your sleep quality and overall well-being. Consistency, environment optimization, and understanding your body's needs are all corner-stones of achieving better sleep despite an erratic work schedule. No matter how unconventional your working hours are, you deserve restorative sleep. Taking these practical steps can pave the path towards better rest and a healthier you.

Managing Jet Lag

Jet lag is an all-too-familiar nemesis for frequent travelers, turning what should be an exciting journey into a foggy experience of sleepless nights and groggy days. The disruption of our natural circadian rhythms by rapid travel across several time zones can leave us feeling out of sync with our surroundings. But don't worry, there's a science-backed approach to managing jet lag that doesn't involve suffering through the symptoms.

First and foremost, understanding what jet lag actually is can make a world of difference. Essentially, it's a temporary sleep disorder resulting from a mismatch between your internal body clock and the external environment induced by crossing multiple time zones. Our bodies have a built-in circadian rhythm—a roughly 24-hour cycle—that regulates sleep and wakefulness, even affecting hormonal release and body temperature. Rapid travel disrupts this rhythm, leading to symptoms such as fatigue, insomnia, poor concentration, and digestive issues (Johns Hopkins Medicine, 2020).

To effectively manage jet lag, one of the most useful strategies begins even before you board your flight. Gradually adjusting your sleep schedule to align more closely with the destination time zone can be remarkably beneficial. For example, if you're traveling east and will lose time, try going to bed an hour earlier for a few days leading up to your trip. Conversely, if you're flying west and will gain time, move your bedtime later (Waterhouse et al., 2007).

Once on the plane, try to simulate the routine of your destination. If it's nighttime there, avoid screens and blue light, and make use of sleep masks to facilitate rest. Conversely, if it's daytime, expose yourself to artificial light or the sun once you arrive. Light exposure is one of the most potent cues for resetting your circadian clock. Strategic light exposure, for approximately 30 minutes to an hour at the right time of the day, can help realign your body's internal clock more quickly (Morgenthaler et al., 2007).

A crucial, yet often overlooked factor in managing jet lag is staying hydrated. Dehydration can worsen the symptoms of jet lag, and the air inside airplanes tends to be particularly dry. Drinking plenty of water before, during, and after your flight ensures your body functions at its best, aiding in quicker recovery and adaptation to new time zones.

Avoiding alcohol and caffeine during your flight can also help manage jet lag, as these substances can interfere with sleep and further dehydrate you (AASM, 2020).

Let's not forget about the impact of food. Consuming meals at the times they would be eaten in your destination can help your body adjust. However, try to eat light meals and avoid heavy, fatty foods, which can be difficult to digest and may disrupt sleep patterns further. Protein-rich foods at breakfast can help promote wakefulness, while complex carbohydrates at dinner may facilitate sleep (Czeisler et al., 2011).

Physical activity also plays a significant role. Engaging in light exercise, such as stretching or walking, upon arrival at your destination can help stimulate circulation and shake off some of the lethargy associated with long flights. A short bout of exercise in the late afternoon or early evening can encourage your body to stay awake longer, aiding in the transition to your new schedule. But, avoid strenuous exercise close to bedtime as it may interfere with your sleep (Youngstedt et al., 2002).

Melatonin, a hormone that regulates sleep-wake cycles, can be an effective tool in managing jet lag. It is naturally produced in response to darkness and helps signal to the body that it's time to sleep. Small doses of melatonin supplements can support your body's adjustment by nudging your circadian rhythm in the right direction. It's generally recommended to take it about 30 minutes before your target bedtime in the new time zone, for up to a few days after arrival (Herxheimer & Petrie, 2002).

Of course, it's always wise to consult a healthcare professional before starting any new supplement. Individual response to melatonin can vary, and it might not be suitable for everyone, particularly those with certain medical conditions or those on specific medications.

Jet lag is inevitable for frequent travelers, but it doesn't have to ruin your trip. Preparation and strategic choices during your journey can go a long way in mitigating its effects. By gradually adjusting your sleep schedule, staying hydrated, managing light exposure, choosing the right foods, incorporating light exercise, and potentially using melatonin, you can reduce the disruptive impact of crossing time zones.

It's about creating a game plan tailored to your needs, flight schedule, and destination. With these tools, you can take back control and make jet lag a thing of the past. The key lies in understanding your body and its rhythms, and making informed choices to support its natural processes. Happy traveling, and even happier sleeping!

Conclusion

Reflecting on the intricate landscape of sleep, it becomes apparent just how integral good sleep is to our overall well-being. We've unpacked the myriad facets that contribute to quality rest, from the biology underpinning our sleep cycles to the influential role of technology and lifestyle choices. Now, as we bring this journey to a close, it's crucial to distill these insights into actionable wisdom that can be practically applied in daily life, reinforcing the transformative power of good sleep for all who seek it.

Why does sleep matter so much? Comprehensive research has shown that poor sleep affects not only day-to-day functioning but also long-term health outcomes. Chronic sleep deprivation can lead to a host of issues, including cognitive impairments, weight gain, and even cardiovascular problems (Walker, 2017). Sleep isn't just a passive state of rest; it's an active process where the brain and body undergo vital repair and regeneration. Knowing this, we need to treat our sleep with the same priority as we do our nutrition and exercise.

Of course, many obstacles stand in the way of achieving the perfect night's rest. Modern life is rife with interruptions and demands that often push sleep to the back burner. But understanding the science behind sleep empowers us to make informed decisions about our nightly rituals and daytime habits. The evidence is undeniable: consistent sleep patterns, mindful technology use, proper nutrition, and regular exercise all play pivotal roles in enhancing sleep quality. By implementing these practices, we set ourselves up for success, both in sleep and in waking life.

One of the most striking revelations is how sleep deprivation compounds over time. It's like a debt that accumulates interest, becoming increasingly harder to repay the longer it goes unchecked. Just as you wouldn't ignore a mounting credit card bill, you shouldn't overlook the significance of mounting sleep debt. Adopting regular sleep schedules and sticking to them even on weekends is a simple yet powerful strategy to prevent this accumulation, debunking the myth that you can 'catch up' on sleep later (Huffington, 2016).

To think about sleep purely in terms of quantity is to miss half the picture. Quality is equally, if not more, important. Engaging in pre-sleep rituals, managing stress through mindfulness practices, and creating an optimal sleep environment are all crucial steps in ensuring that the sleep you do get is restorative. Innovations like blue light blocking glasses and sleep tracking apps have made it easier than ever to monitor and improve our sleep hygiene. Embrace these tools—they're your allies in this essential quest for better sleep.

For many, natural sleep aids can provide a gentle nudge towards better rest, but it's important not to become overly reliant on any quick fixes. Whether it's herbal teas, magnesium supplements, or melatonin, these should be seen as part of a broader strategy rather than standalone solutions. Over-the-counter and prescription sleep aids can be helpful but should always be used under medical guidance to avoid potential side effects and dependencies (Stevenson, 2021).

Now, consider the unique challenges faced by shift workers and frequent travelers who must navigate irregular schedules. Their plight underscores the need for tailored strategies to combat the disruptive impact of these demands on sleep. From adjusting light exposure to syncing with new time zones, there are methods to mitigate these challenges. What's important is that everyone, regardless of their lifestyle constraints, can make meaningful improvements to their sleep patterns with thoughtful adjustments.

A recurring theme in this book is the interconnectedness of different life aspects and their collective impact on sleep. Stress, diet, exercise, and environmental factors all weave together in a complex web. Addressing one area can create a ripple effect that benefits others. This holistic approach reminds us that there's no one-size-fits-all solution, but rather a customizable set of practices that each person can adapt to fit their unique circumstances and needs.

As we close this chapter, let this be your call to action. Consider the small changes you can make starting tonight. Maybe it's setting a consistent bedtime, reducing your screen time before bed, or incurporating a brief meditation session to ease your mind. Remember, optimizing sleep is a journey, not a destination. Every positive change, no matter how minor it may seem, brings you a step closer to the restful, rejuvenating sleep you deserve.

The narrative surrounding sleep is evolving. Once overlooked and undervalued, sleep is now recognized as a cornerstone of health and vitality. This book aimed to demystify the complexities of sleep, providing both the science behind it and the practical tools to improve it. As you go forward, carry these lessons with you. Share them with others. Transform your sleep, and in doing so, transform your life.

In essence, the journey to better sleep starts with awareness and ends with application. You've taken the first step by immersing yourself in the subject matter. Now, it's time to turn that knowledge into action. Prioritize your sleep. Educate others about its significance. Remember that every decision you make throughout the day can have subtle yet profound effects on your sleep quality. Treat your sleep as sacred, and the benefits will ripple across every facet of your life.

Here's to a future marked by restful nights and invigorating days. Sleep well, and live well.

Appendix A:
Appendix

Welcome to the Appendix! In this section, we aim to provide you with practical resources and additional tools to support your journey toward better sleep. This isn't just about tips and tricks; it's about empowering you with the knowledge and resources you need to make meaningful changes. Let's dig into some supplementary materials that will help you optimize your sleep quality effectively.

Resources for Further Reading

If you're keen to dive deeper into the science and practices surrounding sleep, the following books and articles are worth a read:

Why We Sleep by Dr. Matthew Walker - A comprehensive guide on the importance of sleep and how it affects every aspect of our lives.

The Sleep Revolution by Arianna Huffington - This book explores the impact of sleep on our productivity, our happiness, and our physical health, providing practical advice for achieving better sleep.

Sleep Smarter by Shawn Stevenson - A 21-step guide to improving your sleep, which includes actionable tips backed by scientific research.

Peer-reviewed articles can provide you with more detailed scientific insight:

Effects of Sleep Deprivation on Cognitive Performance - This paper discusses how lack of sleep impairs cognitive function (*Doran et al., 2001*).

The Role of Sleep in Emotional Brain Function - This article explains the impact of sleep on our emotional regulation and psychological health (*Walker & van der Helm, 2009*).

Sleep Tracking Tools and Apps

Monitoring your sleep can be a game-changer. Here are some tools and apps that can help you track and improve your sleep quality:

Fitbit - Wearable devices with sleep tracking features that provide insights into your sleep stages, duration, and quality.

Oura Ring - A smart ring that monitors various aspects of sleep, including deep sleep, REM sleep, and overall sleep efficiency.

Sleep Cycle - A smartphone app that analyzes sleep patterns and wakes you up during your lightest sleep phase.

Professional Help and Consultations

Sometimes, the complexities of sleep issues require professional help. Here are some avenues through which you can seek expert advice:

Sleep Clinics - Facilities specializing in diagnosing and treating sleep disorders. They usually conduct sleep studies (polysomnography) to identify and address various issues.

Therapists - Cognitive Behavioral Therapy for Insomnia (CBT-I) is a proven method for treating insomnia and can be facilitated by a licensed therapist.

Nutritionists - Consultation with a nutritionist can provide personalized dietary plans to enhance sleep quality.

Incorporating these resources and tools into your life can significantly enhance your ability to achieve restful and rejuvenating sleep. Remember, the aim is to make consistent, gradual changes that will lead you to a healthier sleep routine and, ultimately, a better quality of life.

Resources for Further Reading

Let's delve into an array of resources that can act as your guides on the journey to deeper, more rejuvenating sleep. These resources will enrich your understanding, clarify your doubts, and offer actionable insights to transform your sleep habits. Whether you're curious about the latest research or you're eager for practical applications, there's something here for everyone.

Unveiling the intricacies of sleep is a lifelong pursuit for many researchers and health professionals. One highly recommended book to kickstart your deeper exploration is "Why We Sleep" by Matthew Walker. This authoritative book walks you through the science behind sleep, its benefits, the consequences of sleep deprivation, and practical tips to improve sleep quality. Walker's clear, engaging style makes complex topics accessible, making it a must-read for anyone aiming to optimize their sleep routine.

For those inclined towards understanding the intersection of lifestyle and sleep, Arianna Huffington's "The Sleep Revolution: Transforming Your Life, One Night at a Time" is a significant read. Huffington illuminates how the sleep epidemic is affecting our health and productivity while offering practical advice to build a robust sleep regimen. Her holistic approach connects sleep quality with overall well-being, providing a roadmap for both personal and professional improvement (Huffington, 2017).

Academic journals offer a wealth of research to those wishing to dive into scientific studies. The journal "Sleep," published by the Sleep

Research Society, covers a wide range of topics from circadian rhythms to the physiological impacts of sleep disorders. It's a valuable resource for professionals and students who want to stay updated on the latest discoveries and developments in sleep science.

For more hands-on guidance, "Sleep Smarter: 21 Essential Strategies to Sleep Your Way to a Better Body, Better Health, and Bigger Success" by Shawn Stevenson provides a mix of scientific information and practical advice. Stevenson's approach is straight-forward and motivational, giving you actionable strategies that can seamlessly integrate into your daily routine. His tips range from optimizing your sleep environment to dietary adjustments for improved sleep.

Additionally, websites such as the National Sleep Foundation (sleepfoundation.org) and the American Academy of Sleep Medicine (aasm.org) are excellent online resources that offer a plethora of articles, research updates, and tips. These organizations provide credible information backed by ongoing research and are frequently updated to include the latest findings in sleep science.

For an academic perspective infused with practical application, Dr. Michael Breus, known as "The Sleep Doctor," has authored multiple insightful guides. His book "The Power of When" explores how understanding your unique biological clock can help you identify the optimal times for critical activities including sleep. Breus' approachable writing helps bridge the gap between scientific research and everyday application (Breus, 2016).

If you're looking for peer-reviewed research articles, platforms like PubMed and Google Scholar are invaluable. Searching for specific keywords such as "sleep disorders," "sleep quality," or "circadian rhythm" can yield a vast array of studies and clinical trials. These resources are particularly beneficial for those seeking in-depth scientific data and statistics.

To better understand sleep disorders, Rustigian et al. (2020) provide comprehensive reviews in their textbook, "Principles and Practice of Sleep Medicine." This textbook is widely used in medical schools and by healthcare professionals to understand the diagnostic and therapeutic nuances associated with various sleep disorders.

Books aren't the only medium to further your sleep education. Podcasts such as "The Model Health Show" hosted by Shawn Stevenson, and "The Matt Walker Podcast" by Matthew Walker, offer engaging discussions on sleep health. These podcasts often feature guest experts and cover a range of topics, offering bite-sized advice you can apply immediately.

For those who appreciate visual learning, TED Talks by sleep experts like Jeff Iliff's "One More Reason to Get a Good Night's Sleep" and Arianna Huffington's "How to Succeed? Get More Sleep," combine compelling storytelling with practical insights. These talks are especially motivational and can be accessed freely online.

Additionally, the "Oxford Handbook of Sleep and Sleep Disorders" is another comprehensive resource that provides an in-depth look into various aspects of sleep, from the basics to advanced concepts. Edited by experts in the field, this handbook covers everything from normal sleep patterns to the complexities of sleep disorders, making it indispensable for any serious student of sleep science (Kushida, 2013).

Lastly, to wrap it up with a newer perspective, consider diving into "The Circadian Code: Lose Weight, Supercharge Your Energy, and Transform Your Health from Morning to Midnight" by Dr. Satchin Panda. His work focuses on the importance of our internal biological clocks and how syncing with them can enhance your sleep quality and overall health. Panda's research offers a different angle by linking circadian health with various lifestyle factors.

These resources aren't just books and articles—they're gateways to better understanding and transforming your sleep. Each offers unique perspectives and actionable advice to help you become a connoisseur of sleep. Let these resources inspire you to dive deeper and perhaps even instill in you a sense of urgency to rectify sleep inadequacies. Because in the end, great sleep isn't just a goal; it's a lifelong investment in your health and well-being.

Sleep Tracking Tools and Apps

The quest for quality sleep has never been more accessible than it is today, thanks to the myriad of sleep tracking tools and apps available in the market. These innovative solutions provide invaluable insights into your sleep patterns, helping you understand and improve your sleep quality. In this section, we'll explore various tools and applications that can assist you in your journey toward better sleep.

One of the most popular categories of sleep tracking tools is wearable devices. These gadgets, often worn on the wrist, like Fitbit or Apple Watch, use sensors to monitor your movements, heart rate, and sometimes even oxygen levels to estimate your sleep stages and duration. Wearables can give you daily updates on how well you slept, providing a sleep score that reflects the quality of your rest. Additionally, many of these devices offer suggestions for improving your sleep habits based on the data they collect.

While wearables provide a wealth of information, they are not the only way to track your sleep. Smartphone apps such as Sleep Cycle and Pillow offer similar functionality without the need for a separate device. These apps use your phone's accelerometer or microphone to track your movements and sounds during sleep. By analyzing this data, they can provide detailed reports on your sleep stages and offer personalized advice for improving your sleep quality.

Some apps go beyond just tracking sleep. For instance, Calm and Headspace not only monitor your sleep patterns but also offer guided meditation and relaxation techniques to help you wind down before bed. These apps can be particularly useful if stress or anxiety is a barrier to getting good sleep. Incorporating mindfulness and meditation into your nightly routine can significantly improve your sleep quality and overall well-being (Kabat-Zinn, 1990).

For those who want a more in-depth analysis, there are advanced sleep tracking systems like the Oura Ring and Whoop Strap. These devices offer a comprehensive look at your sleep, including detailed metrics on sleep stages, heart rate variability, and body temperature. The data is then analyzed to give you a holistic view of your sleep health, including readiness scores that indicate how prepared your body is for the day ahead. Such advanced tracking tools can be especially beneficial for athletes and high-performing professionals who need to optimize every aspect of their physical and mental health.

In addition to these personal devices and apps, some people may benefit from clinical-grade sleep tracking solutions. Polysomnography, for example, is a type of sleep study conducted in a lab setting that uses electrodes to monitor brain activity, eye movements, and other physiological factors. While not practical for everyday use, it can provide a detailed diagnosis for those with severe sleep disorders (Rechtschaffen & Kales, 1968).

Sleep tracking tools are not without their limitations, though. It's essential to understand that these devices and apps provide estimates rather than exact measures of sleep stages and quality. However, they are still incredibly valuable for identifying trends and patterns, which can inform lifestyle changes to improve sleep.

Combining the use of these tools with other strategies, such as creating a conducive sleep environment and maintaining a consistent sleep schedule, can amplify the benefits. Many sleep tracking apps offer integration with other health apps, allowing you to see how factors like exercise, diet, and stress levels impact your sleep. This integrated approach can provide a holistic view of your health and make it easier to identify areas for improvement.

Moreover, sharing your sleep data with a healthcare provider can offer additional insights. Professionals can help you interpret the data in the context of your overall health and recommend targeted interventions. In some cases, they may suggest professional sleep studies or treatments for underlying sleep disorders.

Sleep tracking tools and apps also offer a sense of accountability. Seeing your sleep data in black and white can be a powerful motivator for making necessary changes. Whether it's going to bed earlier, reducing screen time before bed, or making dietary adjustments, having concrete data to back up your decisions can make you more likely to stick with healthy habits.

In conclusion, the myriad of sleep tracking tools and apps available today provide valuable insights into sleep patterns and quality. From wearable devices and smartphone apps to advanced tracking systems and clinical solutions, these tools can help you understand and improve your sleep. While they are not without limitations, the data they provide can be informative and motivating, especially when integrated with other health metrics and professional advice. Embrace these technological advancements as part of your journey to better sleep and overall well-being.

Professional Help and Consultations

Even when you've done everything by the book—optimized your bedtime routine, managed your stress, and even tailored your diet to support sleep—those elusive Z's can still be hard to come by for some. That's where professional help comes into play. It's important to recognize that seeking consultation from a healthcare provider can be a transformative step in your sleep journey.

First and foremost, consulting a primary care physician can be an excellent starting point. They can help identify any underlying medical conditions that might be affecting your sleep. Issues like sleep apnea, chronic insomnia, or restless leg syndrome often require tailored treatments that only a qualified medical professional can provide. Moreover, your primary care physician can offer referrals to sleep specialists or recommend specific therapies that may suit your needs best.

Sleep specialists are usually board-certified physicians who specialize in sleep medicine. These practitioners have the expertise to diagnose and treat a wide range of sleep disorders. They often work in sleep clinics, where they can conduct comprehensive sleep studies to monitor your sleep patterns, breathing, and other physiological parameters during the night. Such evaluations can be crucial in accurately diagnosing issues like obstructive sleep apnea or periodic limb movement disorder, thereby paving the way for effective treatment plans (Epstein et al., 2009).

Behavioral sleep medicine is another avenue worth exploring. This sub-field focuses on the psychological and behavioral aspects of sleep. Cognitive-behavioral therapy for insomnia (CBT-I) is a widely supp-orted, non-pharmacological treatment option that has been proven effective for chronic insomnia. CBT-I involves techniques such as cognitive restructuring, relaxation training, and sleep hygiene edu-cation. A behavioral sleep medicine specialist can guide you through this process, helping to reframe negative thoughts about sleep and cultivate healthier sleep behaviors (Manber et al., 2004).

For those dealing with mental health issues that affect sleep, consulting a psychiatrist or a psychologist can be invaluable. Conditions such as anxiety and depression often have a profound impact on sleep quality. In such cases, addressing the root psychological issues can result in significant improvements in sleep. Medication, talk therapy, or a combination of both may be recommended depending on the severity and nature of your condition. Remember, treating the mental health aspect can sometimes be the key to unlocking better sleep (Harvey et al., 2011).

In many cases, medication may be prescribed as a short-term solution to severe sleep problems. If over-the-counter sleep aids aren't effective, a doctor might recommend prescription medications like benzodiazepines, non-benzodiazepine hypnotics, or melatonin receptor agonists. However, it's crucial to use these medications under close medical supervision because of potential side effects and the risk of dependence.

Don't overlook the role of alternative therapies. Acupuncture, chiropractic care, and even massage therapy can help improve sleep quality for some individuals. Research has suggested that acupuncture, for instance, might help regulate the body's sleep-wake cycle and reduce symptoms of insomnia (Yeung et al., 2009). Holistic approaches to health can complement traditional medical treatments and offer additional avenues to explore.

Sometimes, professional help can also mean working with a dietitian or a nutritionist. Addressing nutritional deficiencies and making dietary modifications can significantly impact sleep quality. A dietitian can provide specific recommendations tailored to your health needs, ensuring that your nutritional intake supports optimal sleep.

If you travel frequently or work irregular hours, specialized consultations can help you manage the unique challenges associated with shift work or jet lag. Strategies like light therapy, melatonin supplementation, or carefully timed naps can be more effective when designed by an expert who understands the intricacies of your lifestyle and work demands (Czeisler, 2015).

Insurance coverage for these consultations and treatments can vary. It's advisable to review your insurance policy or speak with a representative to understand what's covered. Many sleep studies and specialist visits are considered essential and are often covered, but alternative therapies might not be. Being informed about the financial aspect can help you plan your consultations and treatments without unwelcome surprises.

At the end of the day, achieving better sleep often requires a multi-faceted approach. Leveraging professional help ensures that you're not relying solely on trial and error. With expert guidance, you can identify the most effective strategies and interventions tailored to your unique situation. Don't hesitate to make that appointment; investing in quality sleep is ultimately an investment in your overall well-being.

References

Doran, S. M., Van Dongen, H. P. A., & Dinges, D. F. (2001). Sustained attention performance during sleep deprivation: Evidence of state instability. Archives Italiennes de Biologie, 139(3), 253-267. Walker, M. P., & van der Helm, E. (2009). Overnight therapy? The role of sleep in emotional brain processing. Psychological Bulletin, 135(5), 731-748.

Cappuccio, F. P., D'Elia, L., Strazzullo, P., & Miller, M. A. (2010). Sleep Duration and All-Cause Mortality: A Systematic Review and Meta-Analysis of Prospective Studies. Sleep, 33(5), 585-592.

Czeisler, C. A. (1999). The effect of light on the human circadian system. Kodak Codesource Journal, 5(7), 13-23.

Durmer, J. S., & Dinges, D. F. (2005). Neurocognitive consequences of sleep deprivation. Seminars in Neurology, 25(1), 117-129.

Ford, D. E., & Kamerow, D. B. (1989). Epidemiologic study of sleep disturbances and psychiatric disorders. An opportunity for prevention? JAMA, 262(11), 1479-1484.

Grandner, M. A., & Buxton, O. M. (2013). Cardiovascular implications of sleep disorders. Current Biology, 23(16), R689-R693.

Rasch, B., & Born, J. (2013). About Sleep's Role in Memory. Physiological Reviews, 93(2), 681-766.

Roenneberg, T., Allebrandt, K. V., Merrow, M., & Vetter, C. (2012). Social jetlag and obesity. Current Biology, 22(10), 939-943.

Taheri, S., Lin, L., Austin, D., Young, T., & Mignot, E. (2004). Short Sleep Duration is Associated with Reduced Leptin, Elevated Ghrelin, and Increased Body Mass Index. PLOS Medicine, 1(3), e62.

Walker, M. (2017). Why We Sleep: Unlocking the Power of Sleep and Dreams. Scribner.

(Arendt, J. (2009). Managing jet lag: Some of the problems and possible new solutions. Sleep Medicine Reviews, 13(4), 249-256.)

(Saksvik, I.B., Bjorvatn, B., Hetland, H., Sandal, G.M., & Pallesen, S. (2011). Individual differences in tolerance to shift work–a systematic review. Sleep Medicine Reviews, 15(4), 221-235.)

AASM. (2020). Clinical Practice Guideline for the Treatment of Intrinsic Circadian Rhythm Sleep-Wake Disorders. Retrieved from https://aasm.org/clinical-resources/practice-standards/practice-guidelines

Abbasi, B., Kimiagar, M., Sadeghniiat, K., Shirazi, M., Hedayati, M., & Mirlohi, A. (2012). The effect of magnesium supplementation on primary insomnia in elderly: A double-blind placebo-controlled clinical trial. *Journal of Research in Medical Sciences, 17*(12), 1161-1169.

Akhondzadeh, S., Naghavi, H. R., Vazirian, M., Shayeganpour, A., Rashidi, H., & Khani, M. (2001). Passionflower in the treatment of generalized anxiety: a pilot double-blind randomized controlled trial with oxazepam. *Journal of Clinical Pharmacy and Therapeutics, 26*(5), 363-367.

Allen, R. P., Donelson, N. C., Jones, B. C., Li, Y., Manconi, M., Rye, D. B., Winkelman, J. W., & Zucconi, M. (2021). RLS phenotypes: Descriptive evolution and challenges of nosology. Sleep Medicine Reviews, 60, 101522. https://doi.org/10.1016/j.smrv.2021.101522.

Arendt, J., Aldhous, M., & Wright, J. (1997). Synchronisation of a disturbed sleep-wake cycle in a blind man by melatonin treatment. Lancet, 349(9052), 897-898.

Baehr, E. K., Fogg, L. F., & Eastman, C. I. (2003). Intermittent bright light and exercise to entrain human circadian rhythms to night work. American Journal of Physiology-Regulatory, Integrative and Comparative Physiology, 284(3), R714-R722.

Baglioni, C., Battagliese, G., Feige, B., Spiegelhalder, K., Nissen, C., Voderholzer, U., ... & Riemann, D. (2011). Insomnia as a predictor of depression: A meta-analytic evaluation of longitudinal epidemiological studies. Journal of Affective Disorders, 135(1-3), 10-19.

Banks, S., & Dinges, D. F. (2007). Behavioral and physiological consequences of sleep restriction. Journal of Clinical Sleep Medicine, 3(5), 519-528.

Bent, S., Padula, A., Moore, D., Patterson, M., & Mehling, W. (2006). Valerian for sleep: a systematic review and meta-analysis. *American Journal of Medicine, 119*(12), 1001-1009.

Black, D. S., O'Reilly, G. A., Olmstead, R., Breen, E. C., & Irwin, M. R. (2015). Mindfulness meditation and improvement in sleep quality and daytime impairment among older adults with sleep disturbances: A randomized clinical trial. JAMA Internal Medicine, 175(4), 494-501.

Black, D.S., O'Reilly, G.A., Olmstead, R., Breen, E.C., & Irwin, M.R. (2015). Mindfulness meditation and improvement in sleep quality and daytime impairment among older adults with sleep disturbances: A randomized clinical trial. JAMA Internal Medicine, 175(4), 494-501.

Bonnet, M. H., & Arand, D. L. (1992). Caffeine use as a model of acute and chronic insomnia. Sleep, 15(6), 526-536.

Borbély, A. A., Daan, S., Wirz-Justice, A., & Deboer, T. (2016). The Two-Process Model of Sleep Regulation: A Reappraisal. *Journal of Sleep Research*, 25(2), 131-143.

Bravo, J. A., Mattozzi, V., Pearson-Leary, J., & Glaser, P. E. (2013). "Food for thought": The role of nutrition in the modulation of sleep. *Journal of Psychiatric Research*, 47(5), 676-683.

Breus, M. J. (2016). The Power of When: Discover Your Chronotype-- and the Best Time to Eat Lunch, Ask for a Raise, Have Sex, Write a Novel, Take Your Meds, and More. Little, Brown and Company.

Brooks, A., & Lack, L. (2006). A brief afternoon nap following nocturnal sleep restriction: Which nap duration is most recuperative? Sleep, 29(6), 831-840.

Buckley, T.M., & Schatzberg, A.F. (2005). On the interactions of the hypothalamic-pituitary-adrenal (HPA) axis and sleep: Normal HPA axis activity and circadian rhythm, exemplary sleep disorders. Journal of Clinical Endocrinology & Metabolism, 90(5), 3106-3114. https://doi.org/10.1210/jc.2004-1056

Buman, M. P., & King, A. C. (2010). Exercise as a treatment to enhance sleep. American Journal of Lifestyle Medicine, 4(5), 500-514.

Cain, N., & Gradisar, M. (2010). Electronic media use and sleep in school-aged children and adolescents: A review. Sleep Medicine, 11(8), 735-742.

Cajochen, C., Frey, S., Anders, D., Späti, J., Bues, M., Pross, A., & Stefani, O. (2011). Evening exposure to a light-emitting diodes (LED)-backlit computer screen affects circadian physiology and cognitive performance. Journal of Applied Physiology, 110(5), 1432-1438.

Cajochen, C., Munch, M., Kobialka, S., Kräuchi, K., Steiner, R., Oelhafen, P., ... & Wirz-Justice, A. (2006). Evening exposure to a light-emitting diodes (LED)-backlit computer screen affects circadian physiology and cognitive performance. Journal of Applied Physiology, 104(2), 439-447.

Carskadon, M. A., & Dement, W. C. (2005). Normal Human Sleep: An Overview. In M. Kryger, T. Roth, & W. Dement (Eds.), *Principles and Practice of Sleep Medicine*. Saunders.

Carskadon, M. A., & Dement, W. C. (2005). Normal human sleep: An overview. In M. H. Kryger, T. Roth, & W. C. Dement (Eds.), Principles and Practice of Sleep Medicine (4th ed., pp. 13-23). Elsevier Saunders.

Carskadon, M. A., & Dement, W. C. (2011). Normal human sleep: an overview. In M. H. Kryger, T. Roth, & W. C. Dement (Eds.), Principles and Practice of Sleep Medicine (pp. 16-26). Elsevier.

Chang, A. M., Aeschbach, D., Duffy, J. F., & Czeisler, C. A. (2015). Evening use of light-emitting eReaders negatively affects sleep, circadian timing, and next-morning alertness. Proceedings of the National Academy of Sciences, 112(4), 1232-1237.

Chang, A., Aeschbach, D., Duffy, J. F., & Czeisler, C. A. (2015). Evening use of light-emitting eReaders negatively affects sleep, circadian timing, and next-morning alertness. *Proceedings of the National Academy of Sciences*, 112(4), 1232-1237.

Chang, A.-M., Aeschbach, D., Duffy, J. F., & Czeisler, C. A. (2015). Evening use of light-emitting eReaders negatively affects sleep, circadian timing, and next-morning alertness. Proceedings of the National Academy of Sciences, 112(4), 1232-1237.

Chang, A.-M., Aeschbach, D., Duffy, J.F., & Czeisler, C.A. (2015). Evening use of light-emitting eReaders negatively affects sleep, circadian timing, and next-morning alertness. Proceedings of the National Academy of Sciences, 112(4), 1232-1237.

Chang, D. G., Holt, J. A., Sklar, B. C., Groessl, E. J., & Fairbank, J. C. (2016). The effectiveness of yoga for chronic low back pain: A systematic review. Clinical Journal of Pain, 32(2), 181-189.

Conrad, P., & Adams, C. (2012). The effects of clinical aromatherapy for anxiety and depression in the high-risk postpartum woman: A pilot study. Complementary Therapies in Clinical Practice, 18(3), 164-168.

Costello, R. B., Lentino, C. V., Boyd, C. C., O'Connell, M. L., Crawford, C. C., Sprengel, M. L., & Deuster, P. A. (2014). The effectiveness of melatonin for promoting healthy sleep: a rapid evidence assessment of the literature. *Nutrition Journal*, 13(1), 1-16.

Cramer, H., Lauche, R., Langhorst, J., & Dobos, G. (2017). Yoga for depression: A systematic review and meta-analysis. Depression and anxiety, 34(11), 1043-1060.

Czeisler, C. A., Buxton, O. M., & Khalsa, S. B. S. (1999). The human circadian timing system and sleep-wake regulation. In *Sleep medicine: essentials and review* (pp. 1-13).

Czeisler, C. A., Duffy, J. F., Shanahan, T. L., Brown, E. N., Mitchell, J. F., Rimmer, D. W., ... & Kronauer, R. E. (1999). Stability, precision, and near-24-hour period of the human circadian pacemaker. Science, 284(5423), 2177-2181.

Czeisler, C.A. (2013). Perspective: casting light on sleep deficiency. Nature, 497(7450), S13-S13.

Czeisler, C.A., & Buxton, O.M. (2011). The Human Circadian Timing System and Sleep-Wake Regulation. In: Principles and Practice of Sleep Medicine. Philadelphia, PA: Elsevier, 401-417.

Drake, C., Roehrs, T., Shambroom, J., & Roth, T. (2013). Caffeine effects on sleep taken 0, 3, or 6 hours before going to bed. Journal of Clinical Sleep Medicine, 9(11), 1195-1200.

Driver, H. S., & Taylor, S. R. (2000). Exercise and sleep. Sleep Medicine Reviews, 4(4), 387-402.

Ebrahim, I. O., Shapiro, C. M., Williams, A. J., & Fenwick, P. B. (2013). Alcohol and sleep I: effects on normal sleep. Alcoholism: Clinical and Experimental Research, 37(4), 539-549.

Ebrahim, I. O., Shapiro, C. M., Williams, A. J., & Fenwick, P. B. C. (2013). Alcohol and sleep I: effects on normal sleep. Alcoholism: Clinical and Experimental Research, 37(4), 539-549.

Eckel, R. H., King, J. C., Moser, E. A., Griffin, G. E., & Krauss, R. M. (2014). The dietary guidelines for Americans, 2010. Journal of the American Dietetic Association, 112(1), 1643-1650.

Edinger, J. D., Davidson, J. R. T., & Krystal, A. D. (2021). Cognitive behavioral therapy for insomnia in the real world. The Journal of Clinical Psychiatry, 82(5), 30369.

Epstein, L. J., et al. (2009). Clinical guideline for the evaluation, management and long-term care of obstructive sleep apnea in adults. Journal of Clinical Sleep Medicine, 5(3), 263-276.Manber, R., et al. (2004). Cognitive behavioral therapy for insomnia enhances depression outcome in patients with comorbid major depressive disorder and insomnia. Sleep, 27(3), 489-496.Harvey, A. G., et al. (2011). Treating Insomnia in Depression: Insomnia and Depression. Behavior Research and Therapy, 49(3), 181-188.Yeung, W. F., et al. (2009). A systematic review of acupuncture and insomnia. Sleep Medicine Reviews, 13(1), 73-104.Czeisler, C. A. (2015). The Circadian Clock and Human Health. Science, 3(5), 462-465.

Fass, R. (2005). The pathophysiological mechanisms of gastro-esophageal reflux disease and the definition of targeted therapy. Digestive Diseases, 23(1), 18-30.

Fernandez-San-Martin, M. I., Masa-Font, R., Palacios-Soler, L., Sancho-Gomez, P., Calbo-Caldentey, C., & Flores-Mateo, G. (2010).

Effectiveness of Valerian on Insomnia: A Meta-Analysis of Randomized Placebo-Controlled Trials. Sleep Medicine, 11(6), 505-511.

Fernstrom, J. D. (2016). Role of dietary carbohydrates, proteins and fats in the control of food intake and body weight. Vitamins & Hormones, 101, 111-138.

Fernández-San-Martín, M. I., Masa-Font, R., Palacios-Soler, L., Sancho-Gómez, P., Calbó-Caldentey, C., & Flores-Mateo, G. (2010). Effectiveness of Valerian on insomnia: a meta-analysis of randomized placebo-controlled trials. *Sleep Medicine*, 11(6), 505-511.

Garfinkel, D., Laudon, M., Nof, D., & Zisapel, N. (1997). Improvement of sleep quality by melatonin in elderly subjects. Archives of Gerontology and Geriatrics, 24(2), 223-231.

Genzel, L., Spoormaker, V. I., Konrad, B. N., & Dresler, M. (2014). The Role of Rapid Eye Movement Sleep for Amnesia. *Neuroscience & Biobehavioral Reviews*, 49, 105-119.

Gibala, M. J., Gillen, J. B., & Percival, M. E. (2016). Physiological and health-related adaptations to low-volume interval training: influences of nutrition and sex. Frontiers in Physiology, 7, 657.

Glynn, L. (2015). The effects of sugar on sleep quality and duration. Journal of Sleep Research, 24(1), 28-35.

Goldstein, A. N., & Walker, M. P. (2014). The role of sleep in emotional brain function. Annual Review of Clinical Psychology, 10, 679-708.

Gooley, J. J., Chamberlain, K., Smith, K. A., Khalsa, S. B., Rajaratnam, S. M., Van Reen, E., & Czeisler, C. A. (2011). Exposure to room light before bedtime suppresses melatonin onset and shortens melatonin duration in humans. Journal of Clinical Endocrinology & Metabolism, 96(3), E463-E472.

Gunnar, M.R., & Quevedo, K. (2007). The neurobiology of stress and development. Annual Review of Psychology, 58(1), 145-173. https://doi.org/10.1146/annurev.psych.58.110405.085605

Habeeb, A., & Gellai, V. (2020). The impact of spicy foods on sleep quality. Sleep Medicine Reviews, 50, 101254.

Hale, L., & Guan, S. (2015). Screen time and sleep among school-aged children and adolescents: A systematic literature review. Sleep Medicine Reviews, 21, 50-58.

Harmat, L., Takács, J., & Bodizs, R. (2008). Music improves sleep quality in students. Journal of Advanced Nursing, 62(3), 327-335.

Harvey, A. G., & Farrell, C. (2003). The efficacy of a Pennebaker writing intervention for poor sleepers. Behavioral Sleep Medicine, 1(2), 115-123.

Hening, W., Allen, R., Earley, C., & Silber, M. (2017). Restless legs syndrome: A clinical update. National Sleep Foundation. Retrieved from https://sleepfoundation.org/sleep-disorders/more-sleep- disorders/restless legs-syndrome.

Herxheimer, A., & Petrie, K.J. (2002). Melatonin for the prevention and treatment of jet lag. Cochrane Database of Systematic Reviews, (2), CD001520. doi:10.1002/14651858.CD001520

Herz, R. S. (2009). Aromatherapy Facts and Fictions: A Scientific Analysis of Olfactory Effects on Mood, Physiology and Behavior. International Journal of Neuroscience, 119(2), 263-290.

Hirshkowitz, M., Whiton, K., Albert, S. M., Alessi, C., Bruni, O., DonCarlos, L., ... & Adams Hillard, P. J. (2015). National Sleep Foundation's sleep time duration recommendations: methodology and results summary. Sleep Health, 1(1), 40-43.

Hirshkowitz, M., Whiton, K., Albert, S. M., Alessi, C., Bruni, O., DonCarlos, L., ... & Adams Hillard, P. J. (2015). National Sleep

Foundation's sleep time duration recommendations: methodology and results summary. Sleep Health: Journal of the National Sleep Foundation, 1(1), 40-43.

Hirshkowitz, M., Whiton, K., Albert, S. M., Alessi, C., Bruni, O., DonCarlos, L., ... & Ware, J. C. (2015). National Sleep Foundation's sleep time duration recommendations: methodology and results summary. Sleep Health, 1(1), 40-43.

Huffington, A. (2016). The sleep revolution: Transforming your life, one night at a time. Harmony.

Huffington, A. (2016). The sleep revolution: Transforming your life, one night at a time. Harmony.

Huffington, A. (2017). The Sleep Revolution: Transforming Your Life, One Night at a Time. Harmony.

Hwang, E., & Shin, S. (2015). The effects of aromatherapy on sleep improvement: a systematic literature review and meta-analysis. Journal of Alternative and Complementary Medicine, 21(2), 61-68.

Hölzel, B.K., Carmody, J., Vangel, M., Congleton, C., Yerramsetti, S.M., Gard, T., & Lazar, S.W. (2011). Mindfulness practice leads to increases in regional brain gray matter density. Psychiatry Research: Neuroimaging, 191(1), 36-43.

Hülsheger, U. R., Alberts, H. J., Feinholdt, A., & Lang, J. (2013). Benefits of mindfulness at work: The role of mindfulness in emotion regulation, emotional exhaustion, and job satisfaction. Journal of Applied Psychology, 98(2), 310.

Jacobson, B. H., Boolani, A., & Smith, D. B. (2010). Changes in back pain, sleep quality, and perceived stress after introduction of new bedding systems. Journal of Chiropractic Medicine, 9(1), 1-8.

Jacobson, B. H., Boolani, A., & Smith, D. B. (2010). Changes in back pain, sleep quality, and perceived stress after introduction of new bedding systems. Journal of Chiropractic Medicine, 9(1), 1-8.

Johns Hopkins Medicine. (2020). Jet Lag and Travel Sleep Disorders. Retrieved from https://www.hopkinsmedicine.org/health/travel/jet-lag-and-travel-sleep-disorders

Kabat-Zinn, J. (1990). Full Catastrophe Living: Using the Wisdom of Your Body and Mind to Face Stress, Pain, and Illness. Dell Publishing.

Katz, D. A., & McHorney, C. A. (2002). The relationship between insomnia and health-related quality of life in patients with chronic illness. Journal of Family Practice, 51(3), 229-235.

Kennedy, D. O., Wake, G., Savelev, S., Tildesley, N. T. J., Perry, E. K., & Wesnes, K. A. (2006). Modulation of mood and cognitive performance following acute administration of single doses of Melissa officinalis (Lemon balm) with human CNS nicotinic and muscarinic receptor-binding properties. *Neuropsychopharmacology, 31*(9), 1877-1882.

Kolla, B. P., Auger, R. R., & Morgenthaler, T. I. (2018). Diagnosis and management of chronic insomnia. *American Journal of Medicine*, 121(10), 877-884.

Koulivand, P. H., Ghadiri, M. K., & Gorji, A. (2013). Lavender and the nervous system. *Evidence-Based Complementary and Alternative Medicine, 2013*, 681304.

Kredlow, M. A., Capozzol,i M. R., Hearon, B. A., et al. (2015). The effect of physical activity on sleep: a meta-analytic review. Journal of Behavioral Medicine, 38(3), 427-449.

Kuriyama, A., Honda, M., & Hayashino, Y. (2014). Supratherapeutic Doses of Diphenhydramine Are No More Effective than Low Doses for Adult Insomnia: A Two-Stage Crossover Study of Healthy Volunteers. Journal of Clinical Sleep Medicine, 10(4), 353-359.

Lavie, L., Lavie, P., & Herer, P. (2010). Mortality Risk Factors in Obstructive Sleep Apnea: A Coronary Artery Disease Cofactor. Sleep, 33(3), 516-521.

Lewith, G. T., Godfrey, A. D., & Prescott, P. (2005). A single-blinded, randomized pilot study evaluating the aroma of Lavandula angustifolia as a treatment for mild insomnia. Journal of Alternative and Complementary Medicine, 11(4), 631-637.

Lim, J., & Dinges, D. F. (2010). A meta-analysis of the impact of short-term sleep deprivation on cognitive variables. Psychological Bulletin, 136(3), 375-389.

Lin, H. H., Tsai, P. S., Fang, S. C., & Liu, J. F. (2011). Effect of kiwifruit consumption on sleep quality in adults with sleep problems. Asia Pacific Journal of Clinical Nutrition, 20(2), 169-174.

Lockley, S.W., Duffy, J.F., & Czeisler, C.A. (2017). Role of melatonin and its analogs in sleep-promoting effects. In Neurobiology of Sleep and Circadian Rhythms (Pp. 209-224). Academic Press.

Maquet, P. (2001). The role of sleep in learning and memory. Science, 294(5544), 1048-1052.

Mason, M., Welsh, E. J., & Britton, J. (2015). Why do patients not initiate and continue treatment for obstructive sleep apnoea? A systematic review of qualitative research. Sleep Medicine Reviews, 24, 1-11.

Misra, S., & Misra, P. (2015). Effect of acute strength exercise on sleep patterns in male young adults. Sleep Disorders & Therapy, 4(3).

Morgenthaler, T., Alessi, C., Friedman, L., Owens, J., Kapur, V., Boehlecke, B., & Swick, T.J. (2007). Practice parameters for the clinical evaluation and treatment of circadian rhythm sleep disorders. Sleep, 30(11), 1445-1459. doi:10.1093/sleep/30.11.1445

Murphy, P. J., & Campbell, S. S. (1997). Nighttime drop in body temperature: a physiological trigger for sleep onset? Sleep, 20(7), 505-511.

Murphy, P. J., Campbell, S. S., & De Gennaro, T. L. (1997). Nighttime drop in body temperature: A physiological trigger for sleep onset?. Sleep, 20(7), 505-511.

Myllymaki, T., Rusko, H., Syvaoja, H., Juuti, T., Kinnunen, M.-L., & Kyröläinen, H. (2011). Effects of exercise intensity and duration on nocturnal heart rate variability and sleep quality. European Journal of Applied Physiology, 112(3), 801–809.

Myllymäki, T., Rusko, H., Syväoja, H., Juuti, T., Kinnunen, M. L., & Kyröläinen, H. (2012). Effects of exercise intensity and duration on nocturnal heart rate variability and sleep quality. European Journal of Applied Physiology, 112(3), 801–809.

NINDS. (2018). Improving Sleep: A guide to a good night's rest. National Institute of Neurological Disorders and Stroke.

National Sleep Foundation. (2020). Healthy sleep tips. Retrieved from https://www.sleepfoundation.org/articles/healthy-sleep-tips

Ong, J.C., Shapiro, S.L., & Manber, R. (2014). Combining mindfulness meditation with cognitive-behavior therapy for insomnia: A treatment-development study. Behavior Therapy, 39(2), 171-182.

Passos, G. S., Poyares, D., Santana, M. G., Garbuio, S. A., Tufik, S., & Mello, M. T. (2010). Chronic exercise improves sleep and mood in patients with chronic primary insomnia: A randomized clinical trial. Psychotherapy and Psychosomatics, 79(6), 373-379.

Peuhkuri, K., Sihvola, N., & Korpela, R. (2012). Diet promotes sleep duration and quality. *Nutrition Research*, 32(5), 309-319.

Pigeon, W. R., Carr, M., Gorman, C., & Perlis, M. (2010). Effects of a tart cherry juice beverage on the sleep of older adults with insomnia: A pilot study. Journal of Medicinal Food, 13(3), 579-583.

Punjabi, N. M. (2008). The epidemiology of adult obstructive sleep apnea. Proceedings of the American Thoracic Society, 5(2), 136-143.

Rechtschaffen, A., & Kales, A. (1968). A Manual of Standardized Terminology, Techniques, and Scoring System for Sleep Stages of Human Subjects. National Institute of Neurological Diseases and Blindness, Neurological Information Network.

Reid, K. J., Baron, K. G., Lu, B., Naylor, E., Wolfe, L., & Zee, P. C. (2010). Aerobic exercise improves self-reported sleep and quality of life in older adults with insomnia. Sleep Medicine, 11(9), 934-940.

Richardson, G. S., Roehrs, T. A., Rosenthal, L., Koshorek, G., & Roth, T. (2002). Tolerance to Antihistamine Sedative Effects. Sleep, 25(2), 315-320.

Roehrs, T., & Roth, T. (2001). Sleep, sleepiness, and alcohol use. Alcohol Research & Health, 25(2), 101-109.

Roenneberg, T., & Merrow, M. (2015). The circadian clock and human health. Current Biology, 25(10), R432-R437. https://doi.org/10.1016/j.cub.2015.04.011

Roth, T. (2007). Insomnia: Definition, prevalence, etiology, and consequences. Journal of Clinical Sleep Medicine, 3(5), S7-S10.

Sivertsen, B., Hysing, M., Harvey, A. G., & Baker, F. C. (2010). The association between evening intake of caffeinated beverages and sleep in a large sample of adolescents. *Sleep Health*, 18(7), 817-822.

Smith, A. (2002). Caffeine and cognitive performance: A meta-analytic review. Psychological Bulletin, 127(1), 249-259.

Snyder, C. K., & Frühauf, T. (2012). Optimizing sleep health: strategies for sleep hygiene. Journal of Clinical Sleep Medicine, 8(06), 689-696.

Somers, V. K., White, D. P., Amin, R., Abraham, W. T., Costa, F., Culebras, A., ... & Young, T. (2008). Sleep Apnea and Cardiovascular Disease: An American Heart Association/American College of Cardiology Foundation Scientific Statement. Circulation, 118(10), 1080-1111.

Srivastava, J. K., Shankar, E., & Gupta, S. (2010). Chamomile: A herbal medicine of the past with bright future. *Molecular Medicine Reports, 3*(6), 895-901.

Stevenson, S. (2021). Sleep smarter: 21 essential strategies to sleep your way to a better body, better health, and bigger success. Rodale Books.

Stickgold, R. (2005). Sleep-dependent memory consolidation. Nature, 437(7063), 1272-1278.

Stutz, J., Eiholzer, R., & Spengler, C. M. (2019). Effects of evening exercise on sleep in healthy participants: A systematic review and meta-analysis. Sports Medicine, 49(2), 269-287.

Sutherland, K., Vanderveken, O., Tsuda, H., Marklund, M., Gagnadoux, F., Kushida, C. A., ... & Cistulli, P. A. (2014). Oral Appliance Treatment for Obstructive Sleep Apnea: An Update. Journal of Clinical Sleep Medicine, 10(2), 215-227.

Van Cauter, E., Leproult, R., & Plat, L. (2000). Age-related changes in slow wave sleep and REM sleep and relationship with growth hormone and cortisol levels in healthy men. Jama, 284(7), 861-868.

Van Dongen, H. P. A., Maislin, G., Mullington, J. M., & Dinges, D. F. (2003). The cumulative cost of additional wakefulness: dose-response effects on neurobehavioral functions and sleep physiology from chronic sleep restriction and total sleep deprivation. Sleep, 26(2), 117-126.

Venkatraman, V., Chuah, L. Y., Huettel, S. A., & Chee, M. W. (2007). Sleep deprivation elevates expectation of gains and attenuates response to losses following risky decisions. Sleep, 30(5), 603-609.

Walker, M. (2017). Why We Sleep: Unlocking the Power of Sleep and Dreams. Scribner.

Walker, M. (2017). Why we sleep: Unlocking the power of sleep and dreams. Scribner.

Walker, M. (2017). Why we sleep: Unlocking the power of sleep and dreams. Scribner.

Walker, M. P. (2017). Why We Sleep: Unlocking the Power of Sleep and Dreams. Scribner.

Walker, M. P., & Stickgold, R. (2004). Sleep-dependent learning and memory consolidation. Neuron, 44(1), 121-133.

Walters, A. S., Hickey, K., Maltzman, J., Verrico, T., Hening, W. A., Kavey, N., ... & Kohl, R. (1996). A questionnaire study of 138 patients with restless legs syndrome: The 'Night-Walkers' survey. Neurology, 46(1), 92-95.

Waterhouse, J., Reilly, T., & Atkinson, G. (2007). Jet-lag: Trends and coping strategies. The Lancet, 369(9567), 1117-1129. doi:10.1016/S0140-6736(07)60296-5

Watson, N. F., Badr, M. S., Belenky, G., Bliwise, D. L., Buxton, O. M., Buysse, D., ... & Tasali, E. (2015). Recommended amount of sleep for a healthy adult: a joint consensus statement of the American Academy of Sleep Medicine and Sleep Research Society. Sleep, 38(6), 843-844.

Wienecke, L. K., Olesen, J., Oturai, P. S., Ashina, M., & Yoon, M. (2016). Prophylactic and acute treatment of severe nocturnal headache with intravenous magnesium: A

Winbush, N.Y., Gross, C.R., & Kreitzer, M.J. (2007). The effects of mindfulness-based stress reduction on sleep disturbance: A systematic review. Explore: The Journal of Science and Healing, 3(6), 585-591. https://doi.org/10.1016/j.explore.2007.08.003

Wittmann, M., Dinich, J., Merrow, M., & Roenneberg, T. (2006). Social jetlag: misalignment of biological and social time. Chronobiology International, 23(1-2), 497-509. https://doi.org/10.1080/07420520500545979

Wood, L. S., & Reilly, T. (2018). The effect of high-intensity interval training on sleep quality in males and females. Journal of Sports Science and Medicine, 17(4), 569-582.

Youngstedt, S.D., O'Connor, P.J., & Dishman, R.K. (2002). The Effects of Acute Exercise on Sleep: A Quantitative Synthesis. Sleep, 20(3), 203-214.

Zhdanova, I. V., Wurtman, R. J., Regan, M. M., Taylor, J. A., Shi, J. P., & Leclair, O. U. (2001). Melatonin treatment for age-related insomnia. *Journal of Clinical Endocrinology & Metabolism, 86*(10), 4727-4730.

Åkerstedt, T., Kecklund, G., & Axelsson, J. (2007). Impaired sleep after bedtime stress and worries. Biological Psychology, 76(3), 170-173. https://doi.org/10.1016/j.biopsycho.2007.07.010

www.ingramcontent.com/pod-product-compliance
Lightning Source LLC
Chambersburg PA
CBHW052245290526
45785CB00016B/1316